The Bases are Loaded:
A Plan to
BEAT CHILDHOOD OBESITY

By

DAVID CASSLER

Foreword by Keith Clayton, MD

Bases Loaded LLC

The intent of this book is to help individuals with weight management problems. This book is not intended to replace medical guidance. Persons desiring to follow this, or any weight management program should consult with their physician first. Responsibility for any adverse effects resulting from the use of information in this book rests solely with the reader.

Workout Consultant and Cover Art Direction by Spencer Cassler

Instructional Consultant and Graphic Design by Cass Cassler

For more information concerning the Bases Loaded Program, or to order t his book, please contact us or visit us at:

www.beatchildhoodobesityplan.com

Bases Loaded LLC, 592 East 200 North, Orem UT 84097.

Acknowledgments

The author wishes to acknowledge the help received from his brothers, Spencer and Cass, in the creation of this book. Spencer's advice was critical in the early phase of the program, when we were trying to figure out the puzzle pieces of childhood obesity. Without the help of Cass in the publishing phase of this book, there never would have been a book. Many thanks to my dear brothers! Thanks also to my wife and equal partner, Valerie, for her encouragement, love and support. Thanks Joe, for your courage and humor, it made the program fun.

Foreword

By Keith Clayton M.D.

The most important health problem in America today is obesity. Overweight Americans both old and young, are eating their way to a dark future of bad health and serious problems in their daily lives.

Just one example: In America, Type II diabetes has increased 2000% in the past 20 years. Yes, that is right! It is up 20 times what it was when current parents were young children.

This is just the beginning of the problems that will face every overweight person in the future. Here are a few of the other problems that await overweight Americans:

1.   **A much shorter life span**

2.   **A great increase in heart disease**

3.   **A great increase in respiratory and sleep disorders**

4.   **A great increase in emotional challenges like depression and anxiety**

5.   **A great increase in stroke, heart attacks and lung disorders of all kinds.**

I have personally witnessed the havoc and distress caused by obesity in American families. I join those professionals who say that this year, for the first time in 100 years, the average lifespan of an American citizen is going to go down, not up. Obesity is, in my opinion, the leading reason for this dangerous trend.

Illnesses caused by obesity are going to contribute greatly to the financial crisis in health care and to the tremendous increase in emotional illness in America, and the world as a whole. In short, if we do not **DO SOMETHING** about the changes that are causing this national epidemic of overweight families, there will be a **TREMENDOUS PRICE TO PAY.**

I am so proud of the Cassler family for putting this marvelous little book together. They have explained the current problem and given us all many things we can do to "**fix**" the problem for families.

I strongly encourage each parent who is fortunate enough to read this book to **START NOW** making **CHANGES IN LIFESTYLE!** Let us bring families back into the safety of good eating and healthy exercise before it is too late.

May each American take what the Casslers explain to heart. Do it. Do it now. Do it right. Do it right now!

The Casslers have given us the information we need to **PUT THINGS RIGHT**. May we understand and follow their advice.

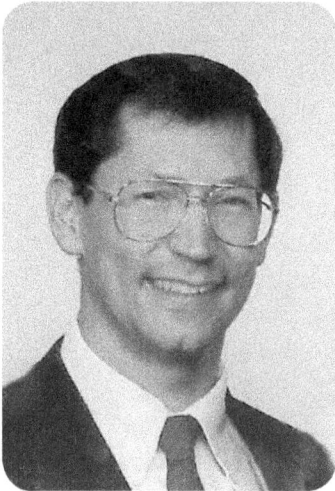

Keith Clayton has been a pediatrician in Utah Valley Utah since 1973. He is currently focusing his pediatric practice on those with ADHD, depression and emotional challenges. He is the father of 8 children and grandfather of 25.

Dedicated to the
Children of the 21st Century

Remember to keep your eye on the ball

Get up quickly if perchance you fall

For you have a date with destiny to meet

God grant power to your arms and swiftness to your feet

Run the bases strong and true

And let the world stand back and wonder at the miracle of you

David Cassler

Table of Contents

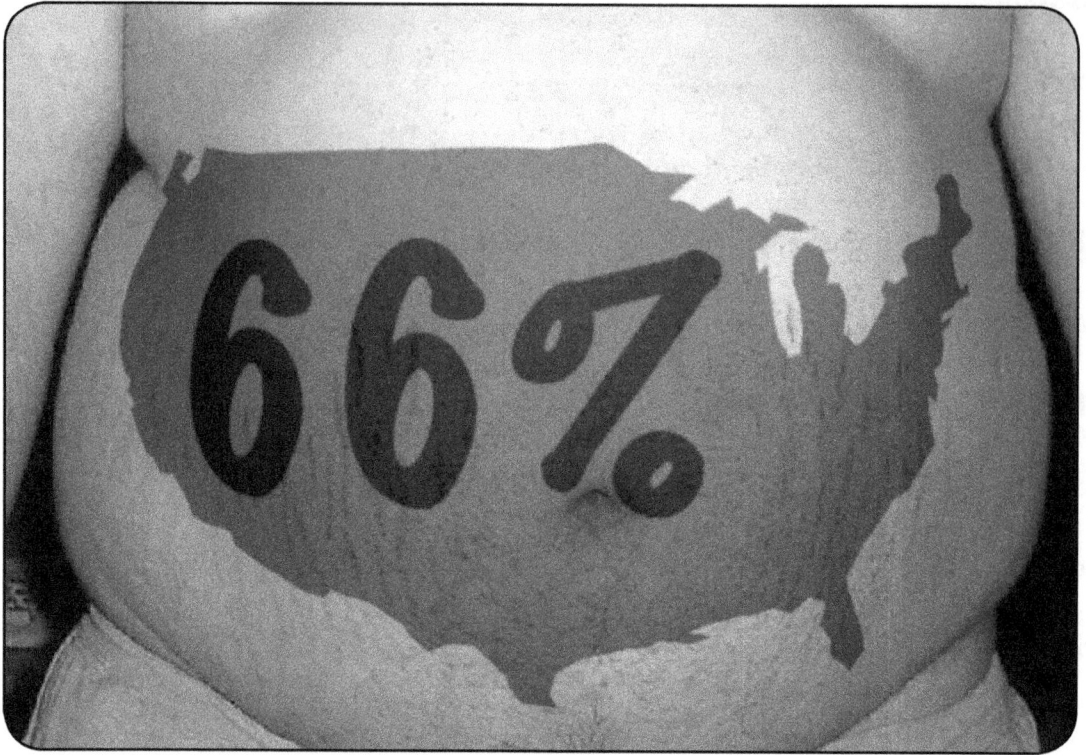

Two-thirds of Americans are either overweight or obese, and the average American today is 23 pounds overweight ...[1]

Introduction

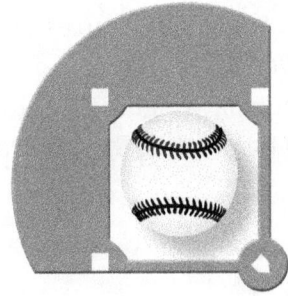

Childhood obesity and diabetes have become chronic problems in America and other developed nations of the world. A recent news article maps out a very sobering profile of the challenges America faces regarding this epidemic.

Obesity, and with it diabetes, are the only significant health problems that are getting worse in this country, and they are getting worse rapidly ... it is not an individual problem but a societal problem—as the nation's health bill illustrates—that will take society—wide efforts to reverse ... diabetes costs the nation $190 billion a year to treat, and excess weight is the single biggest risk factor for developing diabetes ... obese diabetics are the hardest to treat, with higher rates of foot ulcers and amputations, among other things.[2]

Contrast the Bad News with the Good

What is this we hear, some good news in the midst of this epidemic? Yes! The good news has arrived in the form of a little book, this small book! "The Bases are Loaded" refers to a situation in baseball, where the team that is up to bat has a runner on each of the three bases. The bases are thus full or loaded. It is a particularly good position to be in, for the team that is at bat.

Why is it a good situation? If the bases are loaded then, the next batter has the potential to get a hit and provide teammates on base the opportunity to score. The best possible thing that could happen would be for the batter to get a home run, which would allow all three teammates and the batter to score. This special home run is a "grand slam." It does not happen very often in the game of baseball, but when it does happen, it remains an unforgettable experience for all who attend it.

We can compare America's obesity epidemic to this "bases loaded" situation. The good news is that we, those of us who are overweight or obese, are the side that is up to bat! The bases are not only full, but they are "loaded" with some very heavy players.

Below are a few pictures of a former player, my son, Joe Cassler. The weight loss that Joe achieved in the course of one year amounted to 28% of his body weight. This is comparable to a person weighing 200 pounds losing 56 pounds, or a person weighing 300 pounds losing 84 pounds. Even more remarkable, Joe lost this weight when he was 12 years old.

Slim

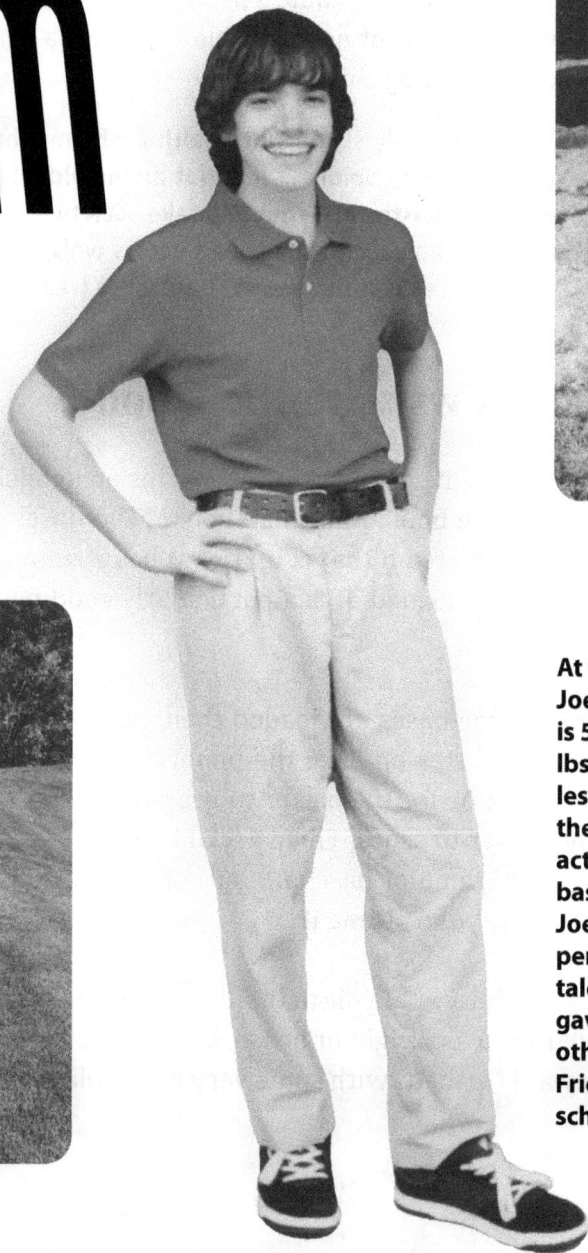

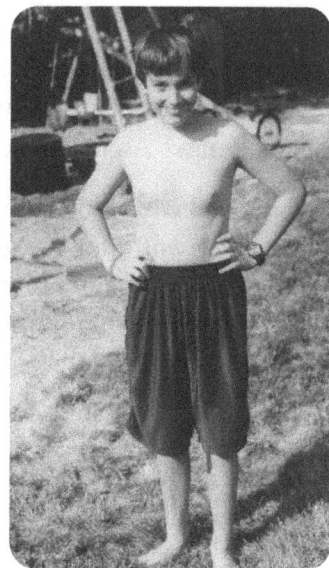

September 2006

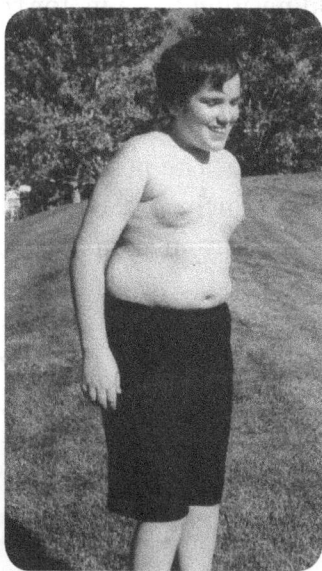

October 2005

At the writing of this book, Joe is fifteen years old. He is 5'11" and weighs 125 lbs., which is 18 pounds less than he weighed at the age of 11. His favorite activity is no longer baseball, but rather music. Joe is a good-hearted person that has musical talent. Joe's music teacher gave him a nickname that others have picked up. Friends around the music school call Joe "Slim."

Hope

In America's bases loaded situation, there is hope in the eyes, and hearts of those on base, and a feeling in the air that the time might be right for the unforgettable to happen. The next player needs to step up to the plate, swing their bat strong and true, and connect with the ball solidly so that we might run the bases and win this deadlocked game.

Who will be this mighty batter, and when will they come to bat? I believe that the mighty player could be your son or daughter. My son, Joe came to bat four years ago when he was eleven and twelve years old. At that time, 45% of his body weight was fat. This book is about Joe's time at bat and what he did to achieve healthy weight. Because of the things Joe accomplished, I think there will be many mighty batters to come.

Who is this Book for?

This book is admittedly not for everyone. There are good weight management programs available that will give faster results than the Bases Loaded Program. According to statistics, about one out of three Americans do not have a weight problem. To those Americans that do not have a problem we say, "Keep up the good work, keep doing what you are doing." There remains another two thirds of America that have weight problems. Children, parents, and students are overweight. People that hold "nine to five" jobs, those who are subject to the class bells, whistles, and time clocks that set the pace for America need a workable plan.

It is About the Future

If there are good weight management programs out there that offer faster results, why should a family consider the Bases Loaded Program? Unfortunately, the few good programs out there are oriented to adults.

The Bases Loaded Program specifically addresses the needs, schedule, and psychology of a child. Childhood is a time where "change" is the rule of the day. Children are changing physically, intellectually, and emotionally at an accelerated pace. Fast results, in the realm of weight loss, require abrupt changes in lifestyle. Frankly, children cannot handle such abrupt changes and still do all the other things that they are required to do.

Added to this, a child or teenager's mind is keenly aware of their environment. They fear failure in school and rejection from their peers. In connection with this idea, an overweight or obese child has had experience with failure. Let us once again use a metaphor from baseball to gain greater insight into the minds and hearts of children.

When a child comes up to bat against obesity, it is like a new player from the minor league facing a pitcher in the major league for the first time. I will call this new player, "Rookie." Rookie's opponent, "Obesity" is a seasoned pitcher. Obesity delivers three pitches in quick order, a fastball, a curve, and a changeup pitch. All three of these pitches confound Rookie. He swings and misses all three pitches. He strikes out and feels humiliated and discouraged. He goes to bat a few more times in the course of the game, but each time is the same—another strikeout. By the end of the day, Rookie wants to give up, crawl under a rock, and never play the game of baseball again.

Fortunately, he has an understanding coach. After the game, the coach encourages Rookie not to give up. He says; "Look, you have just faced the toughest professional pitcher in the big leagues. This guy is unpredictable, but not unbeatable! I know we can figure him out. We have expert coaches on our staff. We will study the game films and see what he is doing in his pitching. We will coach you on your batting. Keep your head up, kid, we will beat this guy!"

Hopefully this little story shows the need for intervention. Children that are dealing with weight problems need to know that their foe is beatable. This book is about the future. It is about the future of children! Obesity is an unmerciful taskmaster that whispers words of discouragement and failure into the minds and hearts of children. The Bases Loaded Program builds confidence within children. Children succeed in overcoming a tremendous obstacle, and success becomes a pattern for them, a new way of life!

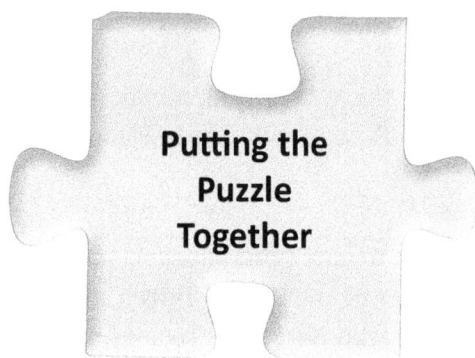

Putting the Puzzle Together

The plan to beat childhood obesity is like a puzzle that is only partially put together. We have "expert coaches," researchers and professionals, who have figured out puzzle pieces. With every puzzle, there is always an overlooked piece that gets lost in the shuffle of things. In this book, we are going to search every corner of the ballfield for those missing pieces and find them!

We have experiences from life that will help us understand the opponent. Children have understanding coaches, parents who will encourage them by walking the same path that they do. We have most of the pieces, and the resolve to find the missing pieces. We need only to start putting the puzzle together. That is what this book is all about. We are going to put the obesity puzzle together and develop a plan to beat childhood obesity!

The Bases Loaded Theory and the Hunter/Gatherers

Many overweight children lead physically active lives. This has led some to believe "genetics" plays the greatest role in obesity. While I do not discount the role genetics plays in childhood obesity, the premise of this book discounts the notion that genetics is the primary factor causing obesity in youth. It is within the environment of the family that obesity begins. I believe that childhood obesity begins with poor nutrition, and a hectic lifestyle that revolves around the time clock and convenience. If this premise is true, then a child need not be doomed to an uncontrollable fate of obesity. Healthy weight is attainable! Through understanding and implementation of the principles contained in this book, both parents and children will gain a new measure of empowerment. They will experience the indescribable joy of being able "to act," rather than "be acted upon."

While I believe "genetics" is not the primary factor causing obesity, the "Bases Loaded" theory agrees with scientific evidence that there is a "genetic condition" that plays a crucial role in the incidence of childhood obesity.

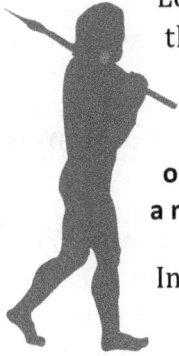

"Even though our ancestral line diverged from the chimpanzees more than four million years ago, for example, there is only a 1.6 percent difference between our present genetic makeup and that of humans who lived during the Paleolithic era, a mere 40,000 to 15,000 years ago, is believed to be negligible." [3]

In terms of "genetic programming" human beings are "hardwired" like the earliest of human-like creatures. We commonly refer to these creatures as cavemen and their descendants as hunter/gatherers. What significance does this scientific fact have in terms of the incidence of modern obesity?

Think of it this way; Americans, biologically speaking, can be compared to hunter/gatherers that have been transported in a time machine to truly unnatural surroundings. The "lifestyle" that we have been programmed for has been taken away from us, and we are now living in a way that is foreign to the biological core of human beings.

How did the hunter/gatherers live? Most people have gone camping in the wilderness for a few days, and can relate to the term "roughing it." Imagine a camping experience without sleeping bags, tents, store bought food, flashlights, clothes, and every other camping convenience. Imagine that such a camping experience were not for just a few days, but for an entire lifetime. Such are the conditions for which we are programmed. In other words, human beings are hardwired for survival.

It Starts at Home

If indeed, it is within the environment of the family that childhood obesity occurs, it makes sense that the family becomes the best support group for undoing the problem. This book is for families. In particular, we have oriented it to parents because they hold the key to unraveling the obesity problem.

The program requires the cooperation of at least two family members—a parent and a child—in order to be successful. It goes without saying that the person doing the program must truly want to do the program. A person cannot be forced to change. That desire has to come from within the person. Just as important is the cooperation that must come from the family members who buy and prepare the meals.

A Practical and Positive Program

Parents will be happy to know that the program discussed in this book will make life a lot less complicated and less expensive in the long-term.

New research shows medical spending averages $1,400 more a year for an obese person than for someone with normal weight. [4]

The Bases Loaded Program will increase the health and vitality of your family. With a healthy family, medical bills will be lower. The plan advocates a return to eating nutritiously. Believe it or not, a person who orients their spending dollars with nutrition in mind will save money over those who get their food with convenience in mind. Thus, the Bases Loaded Program is both a practical and long range means to save money.

The Bases Loaded Program is not a bodybuilding program. It is not a quick fix or a crash course. Rather, it is a weight loss program that helps parents and children get rid of excess fat, and achieve "an ideal" or "healthy" weight. Even more than the physical aspect of the program, Bases Loaded is a book about making positive changes in life. The Bases Loaded Program requires lifestyle changes, a new way of doing things. It thus is a collection of principles that have the ability to stay with family members a lifetime. It is a program that requires patience. The dates on the "before and after" photographs presented earlier span a year's time.

The physical changes that accompanied Joe's weight loss over this period were imperceptible to those who saw Joe on a day-to-day basis, but, in the words of a visiting relative who had not seen Joe during the period of these two photos, "I would not have recognized him as Joe, had I passed him on the street!"

While the outward changes were slow, the inward changes Joe experienced were immediate and recognizable. Shortly after starting the program, Joe expressed himself in phrases such as, "I feel better," or, "This is awesome!" It is this potential for inward change, which makes the Bases Loaded Program worth the effort. The principles outlined in this book have the ability to give one a sense of "well-being" from the very start. As one feels better physically, it is only natural that feelings of confidence and peace follow.

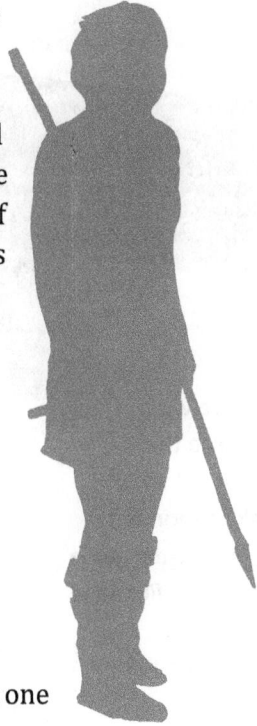

Potential Benefits

Here are some of the benefits Joe experienced, and possibilities that one may experience from this program, as well.

- **Eat just as much food as before, but eating habits will be modified**

- **A sense of satisfaction from eating without feeling a compulsion to overeat**

- **Taste of food - better**

- **Increased energy, vitality**

- **Improved ability to focus on work or school work, activities requiring mental effort**

- **Feel less stress**

- **Sleep improvement**

- **Slow and safe weight loss**

- **Increased love and appreciation for other family members**

- **Look better, laugh more and be complemented by others.**

Joe's Reflections

Before we get into the book, let us take a moment and consider some of Joe's reflections about the Bases Loaded Program.

I started to gain weight when I went into the 4th grade. I began to notice that my friendships with everyone at school, were not the same as when I was younger (when I was on the "fit list"). My thoughts were focused on my pleasure, which was junk food. I cared more for tasty food than my friendships at school.

In the condition that I was, friends were surprised if I made a goal in soccer. As I look back, I realize that this fact hurt my feelings as much as their cheers of encouragement lifted my spirits. I knew that something was wrong when everyone in my PE-class could run faster than me. When they finished, they cheered for me. Seeing how far ahead they were, I regarded the cheers as taunts.

I was frustrated. While I exerted all my effort, I would see others doing a lot more push-ups and sit-ups without breaking a sweat. In PE-class, they divide everyone into three ranks of fitness: Presidential, National, and Participant. As you might guess, I always was in the Participant category. After 5 years of this, it broke my heart. I literally burst into tears, because I felt that I was not good enough, and no one could expect much from me physically.

I also struggled to understand concepts in school. Everyone seemed to understand things that I could not understand. This affected me almost as much as my physical disadvantages.

In 6th grade, I began homeschool. I started exercising with my dad and eating better. At first I was reluctant to do this program, but I soon changed my mind.

After losing 20-25 pounds, I looked in the mirror and noticed that I started to look like my friends: fit. I got excited. I started to like exercising, and lost 15 more pounds of weight. My dad gave me a new life. When I see pictures of when I was overweight, I always say to myself, "That is another person." Now when I look into the mirror, I never see that person. With the changes I have been through I have never had anyone taunt me again.

I am now going to high school and learning how to drive. I made the high honor roll last year (dad told me to say that) and enjoy the different things that I am doing in school, sports and guitar.

Suggestions on How to Read this Book

We encourage readers to read this book twice. Concentrate on the narrative and accompanying visuals during your first reading. The narrative is a simple explanation of the Bases Loaded theory and method from a parent's perspective. It should be noted here that I am the main meal maker of the household. I also run my own business from home. Thus, I was able to be with Joe and experience what he experienced, day in and day out. The narrative constitutes "a writing" from the heart. It is the "game film," what Joe and I experienced physically, in Joe's battle against obesity.

Concentrate on the supplemental writings during your second reading. These are supporting references from the experts written in bold print. Once again, refer to the visual images along with the words of the experts. At the end of each chapter, check your knowledge by answering some questions that will help reinforce the principles just taught. Together the writings and activities help one put the childhood obesity puzzle together piece by piece. When the puzzle comes together, and the large picture emerges, we hope that parents will desire to implement these principles into family life.

Any sports analyst will say that it is easy to comprehend the working mechanics of a game, but to gain a real understanding of the game, one must play the game. That is the only way to gain an "understanding of the heart," and it is only through an "understanding heart" that the battle against childhood obesity can be won.

Finally, it must be stated that this program for achieving ideal weight is recommended as a preventative measure. It is a method to prevent a weight problem from becoming a serious problem. As part of the Bases Loaded Program, we recommend that all parents and children consult with their respective doctor before implementing this, or any, weight management program.

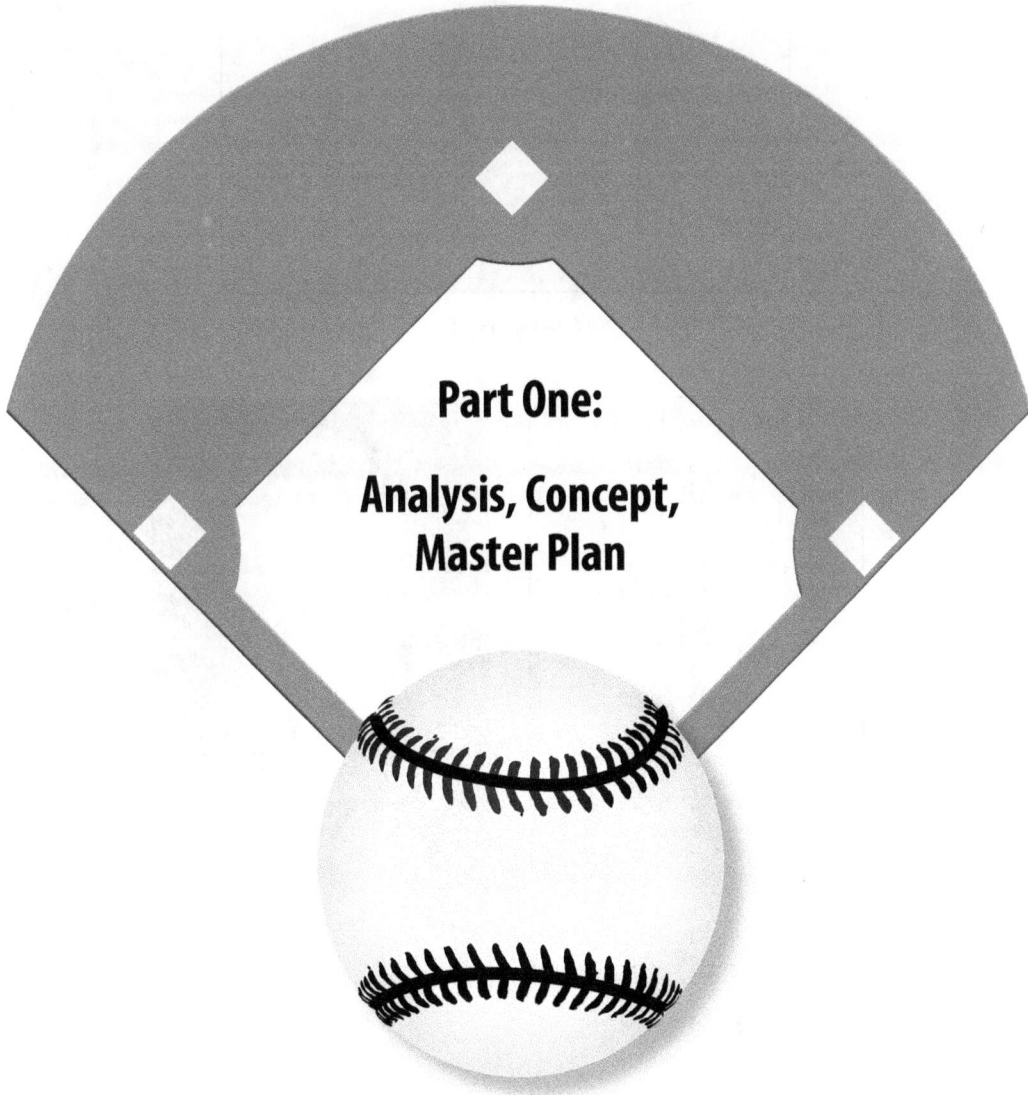

Part One:

Analysis, Concept, Master Plan

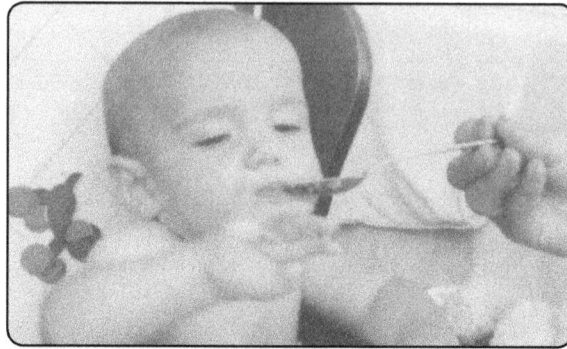

1 year old

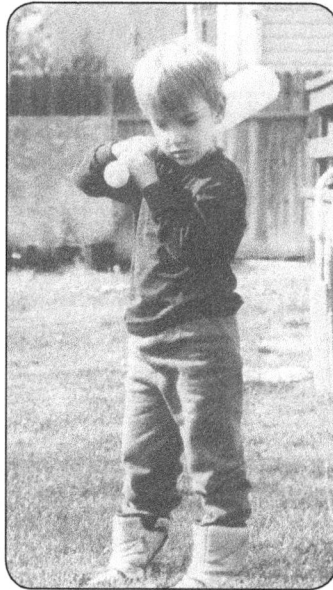

4 years old

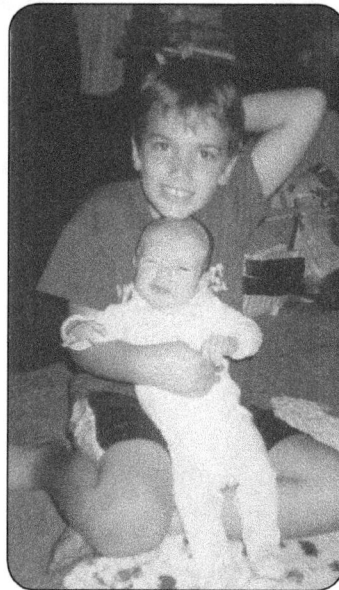

8 years old

Despite our doctor's good advice and our good intentions, we lacked the commitment to implement a plan of action.

Joe's Short History

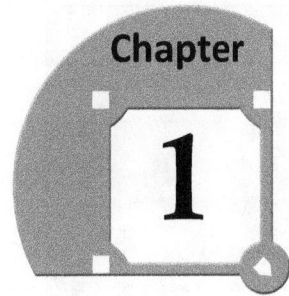

Chapter

1

He was a skinny kid when he was a little boy. His mom used to call him "String Bean." Joe was always active as a child. He loved to swing the plastic bat and could hit the plastic ball over the back yard fence when he was 4 years old.

As parents, we saw the athletic potential he possessed and enrolled him in T-ball, soccer, and hockey. Joe's eating habits seemed normal. When he started kindergarten and had to get up early, he would not eat a big breakfast. He attended a private school that did not provide hot lunch. Lunch meals were out of the lunch box.

When Joe arrived home from school, he made up for his lack of appetite during the morning. His favorite snacks were carbohydrates such as chips, noodles, cereal, and candy. Juice was his drink of choice.

Joe ate the parts of dinner he liked. His favorites were carbohydrates such as pasta, mashed potatoes, French fries, pizza and fast food. Joe always seemed to be hungry within an hour after eating dinner, and would satisfy this hunger by eating more snacks. It seemed that Joe ate more snack food than food from his meals.

Joe usually finished his homework early. Hockey practice occurred one night a week. Joe spent the other nights in front of the TV watching videos. Snacks continued till bedtime. We noticed that, after the summer of second grade, Joe appeared a little heavy. My fears dissipated during third grade when Joe slimmed down again, but when Joe started fourth grade he somehow appeared heavier than the summer previous. I calmed my wife's fears by saying; "He will slim down as he did last year."

Fourth grade was a hard year for Joe. He seemed to lose confidence in the classroom. He continued to be active in sports, but this time he failed to slim down.

Joe and his three brothers visited the family doctor for their annual check-up as Joe was about to enter 5th grade. At that time, the family doctor advised us, "Joe should lose about 10 pounds."

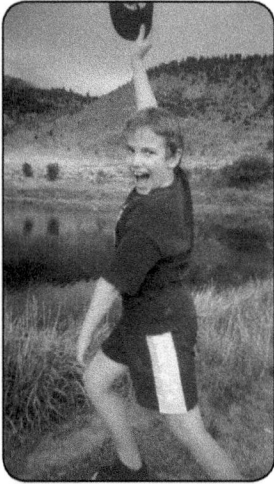

9 years old

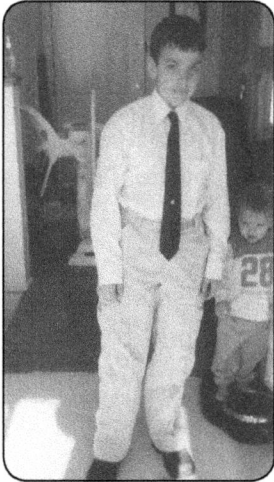

10 years old

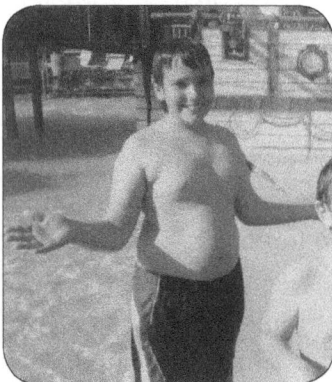

11 years old

He told us that if Joe continued to gain weight in his torso region, that pretty soon his body would start producing the hormone estrogen and that this would in turn accelerate weight gain and delay puberty.

Despite our doctor's good advice and our good intentions, we lacked the commitment to implement a plan of action. As the year progressed other family matters took priority. Joe was enjoying his 5th grade teacher and doing well in school.

He continued to play hockey and was always happy around the house. The only thing we implemented concerning Joe's weight problem was to have him stop snacking an hour before bedtime.

When summer arrived, we had a disheartening experience. It was Joe's first baseball game of the year. He hit the ball second time up to bat and tried running to first base. The rolls of fat that were hidden under hockey equipment all winter bounced up and down with every stride. Instead of losing 10 pounds over the course of the year, Joe had gained another 15 pounds.

My wife and I changed priorities. We began to read books about nutrition. Prior to this, we were considering home-schooling Joe for the coming year. During the course of the season, we became excited about the prospect of teaching Joe at home and using the upcoming year to help him lose weight.

With the help of my brother Spencer, Joe's uncle, we began implementing a strategy in the fall of 2005. The plan evolved over the course of the next few months. The "Bases Loaded Program" (BL-Program), or "Bases Loaded Plan" (BL-Plan), finally emerged in the spring of 2006.

Physical Activity Triangle

In this book, we will use some simple visual models to help us understand the complexities of childhood obesity. These models will employ geometric shapes to represent certain activities or processes that the human body performs.

We will use the shape of a triangle **(Figure 01)**, to represent the physical activity of the body. Physical activity includes exercise or any physical exertion that compels the human body to move. Since work or exercise requires the body to expend energy, we will distinguish this triangle from other triangles in the book, by rendering it with a light shade. Thus, we call the light shaded triangle the Physical Activity Triangle (PA-Triangle).

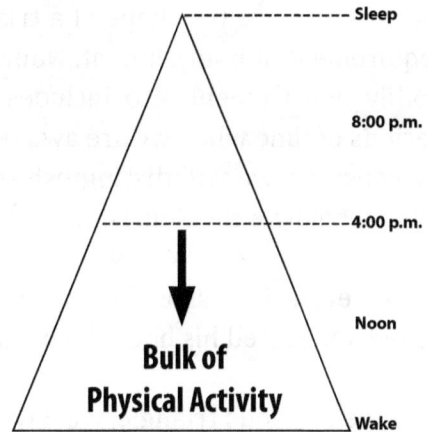

Figure 01: The Physical Activity Triangle - Joe did most of his physical activities in the morning and afternoon hours before 4:00 p.m.

Let us examine Joe's short history. We will use the PA-Triangle to help us understand how Joe worked his body in a typical day prior to implementing the program.

Notice that we have introduced the concept of time into the visual representation. In a typical day, Joe woke up and did most of his physical activities in the morning and afternoon hours. We represent these physical activities by the part of the PA-Triangle underneath the dashed line marked "4 p.m."

We see the amount of physical activity Joe accomplished in the evening represented by the portion of the PA-Triangle above the dashed line. Analysing the two areas, we see that the amount of physical activity performed in the evening is relatively small compared to the physical activity done in the morning and afternoon.

Try drawing your own physical activity triangle and compare it to Joe's. Do not be surprised if it looks the same. Most students and workers are physically active in the morning and afternoon. Exercise conscious professionals tend to wake up early, and do their workout before starting the workday. Evening and nights usually mean a tapering off of physical activity, a time to relax the body. Now let us look at another triangle.

The Nourishment Triangle

We will also use the shape of a triangle **(Figure 02)**, to represent the human body's daily requirement of nourishment. Nourishment includes the consumption of food and drink. Bodily nourishment also includes the need for rest. By rest, we are referring to the periods of time when we are awake but not active. Since food is a tangible substance that we consume, we will distinguish this triangle with a dark shade. Thus, we call the dark shaded triangle the Nourishment Triangle (N-Triangle).

Let us review Joe's short history. We will use the N-Triangle to help us understand how Joe fueled and rested his body during a typical day before his program.

Like the previous triangle, we have introduced the concept of time into the visual image. In a typical day, Joe woke up, got a quick bite to eat and rushed off to the days activities. The smallest part of the N-Triangle points downward and falls in the "before noon" period. The greatest portion of the N-Triangle is above the dashed line marked 4 p.m., and represents the food Joe consumed as well as the rest he received during the late afternoon and evening hours.

Compare your own N-Triangle to Joe's. Most students and workers have N-Triangles that look like his. If we work all morning and afternoon, it is only natural that we rest and refuel in the evening.

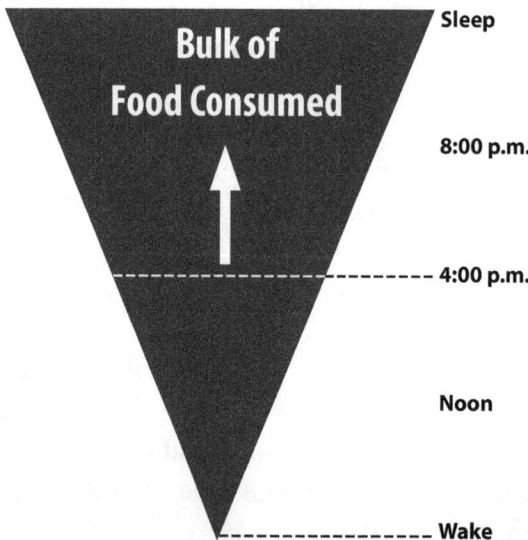

Figure 02: Nourishment Triangle—Joe consumed the bulk of his food during the evening hours between 4:00 p.m. and when he went to sleep.

✔ Check Your Understanding

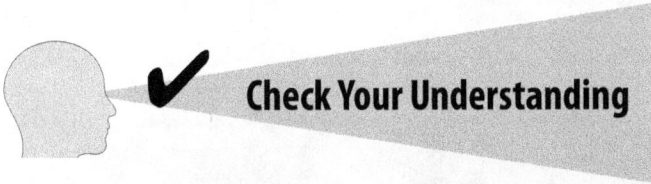

1. **Did Joe do most of his physical activities before or after 4:00 p.m?**

    Answer: *Joe did most of his physical activities before 4:00 p.m.*

2. **Did Joe eat most of his daily food before or after 4:00 p.m?**

    Answer: *Joe received most of his daily food after 4:00 p.m.*

3. **What were Joe's favorite types of food?**

    Answer: *Joe's favorite types of food were carbohydrates such as pizza, noodles, chips, fries and candy.*

4. **Did Joe seem to eat more food during his meals, or during snacks?**

    Answer: *Joe seemed to eat more during snacks compared to the food he ate during meals.*

5. **What were Joe's daily physical activities?**

    Answer: *Joe's physical activities during a typical school day included recess, walking to classes, and the physical exercise he received in physical education class.*

6. **What was the orientation of Joe's PA (Physical Activity)-Triangle, A or B?**

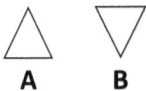

    △ ▽
    A   B
    Answer: *A*

7. **What was the orientation of Joe's N (Nourishment)-Triangle, A or B?**

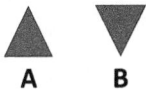

    ▲ ▼
    A   B
    Answer: *B*

The period of time between waking up, and going to sleep, is a period of time where our metabolism is constantly changing its rate of fuel consumption.

The Bases Loaded Concept

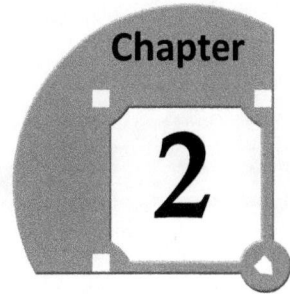

Chapter

2

The concept behind the Bases Loaded Program is truly simple. We will switch the orientation of the Physical Activity Triangle. The Bases Loaded Program advocates doing most physical activity in the evening, rather than the morning.

We will also switch the orientation of the Nourishment Triangle. The Bases Loaded Program advocates receiving the bulk of food and physical rest in the morning, rather than the evening.

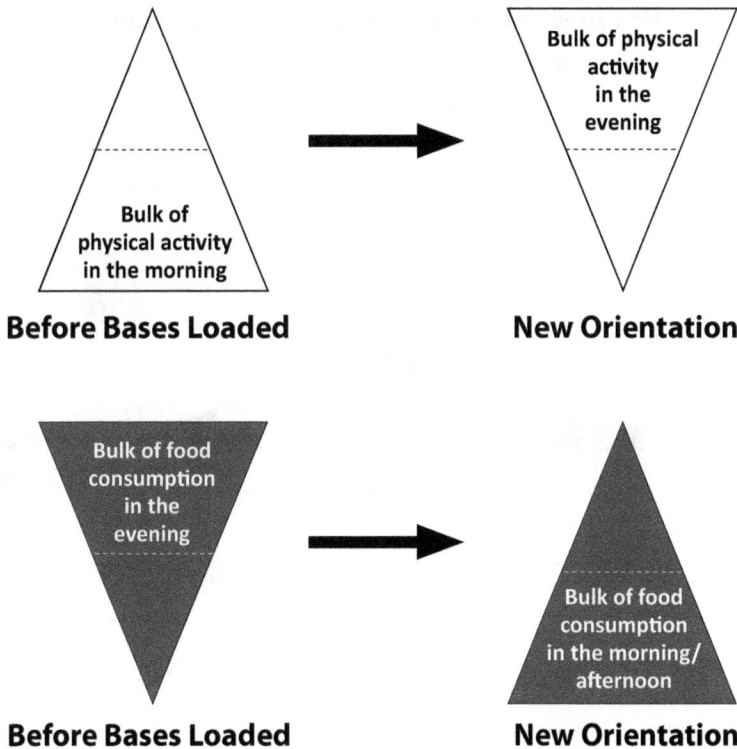

Bulk of
physical activity
in the morning

Before Bases Loaded

Bulk of physical
activity
in the
evening

New Orientation

Bulk of food
consumption
in the
evening

Before Bases Loaded

Bulk of food
consumption
in the morning/
afternoon

New Orientation

Figure 03: Bases Loaded Concept - The Bases Loaded program advocates eating the bulk of your food in the morning, and doing the bulk of your physical activity in the evening.

The Metabolism Diamond

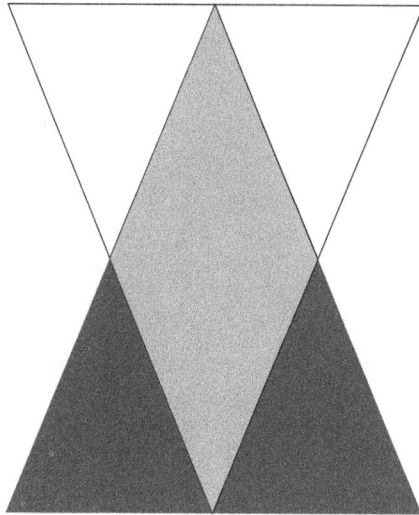

Key player in the Bases Loaded Program

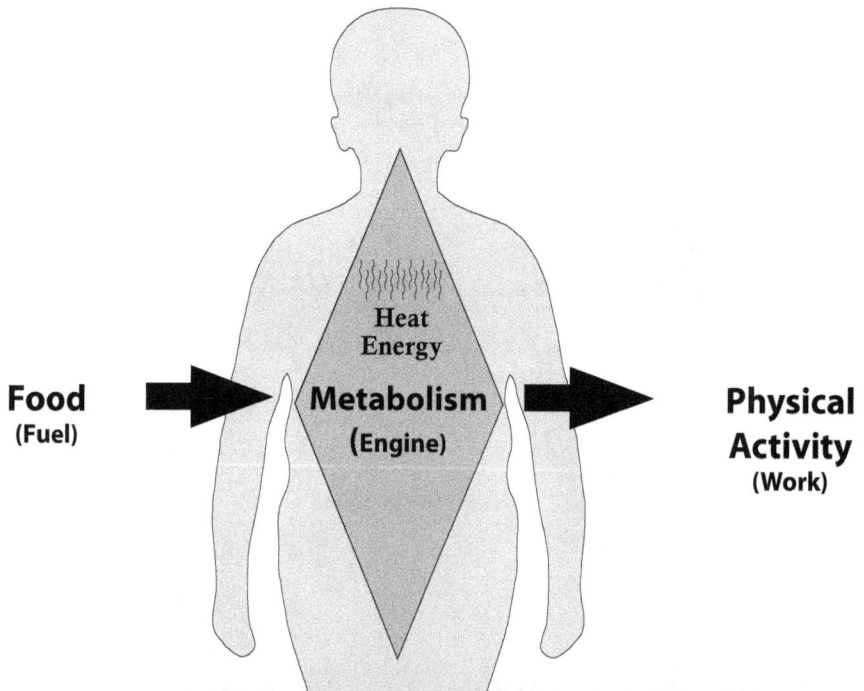

Heat Energy

Food
(Fuel)

Metabolism
(Engine)

Physical Activity
(Work)

Figure 04: The Metabolism Diamond - Metabolism is the body's system, for converting food into energy. We can compare metabolism to an engine of a car.

The Metabolism Diamond

If we were to overlap the new triangles **(Figure 04)**, we would find that the dark shade and light shade combine to create a medium shaded diamond. Surrounding the diamond are four triangles, two dark on the bottom, and two light shaded triangles on the top. To understand why we have reoriented the triangles, we need to gain an understanding of the medium shaded diamond.

The medium shaded diamond is an abstraction for a very real process or phenomenon within the human body. "Metabolism" is the medium shaded diamond and a key player in the Bases Loaded Program. As the overlapping triangles suggest, metabolism transforms food into energy, which in turn, allows the body to do physical work.

In upcoming models, we will represent metabolism by using a few triangles connected together to create an interesting geometric shape. This geometric shape will vary from model to model, according to the variables of work and food that we will consider for each respective model. For convenience sake, we will sometimes refer to the medium shaded shape as the "Metabolism Diamond."

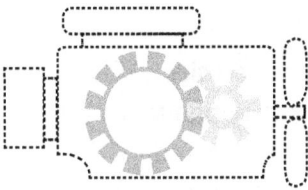

The Inward Engine

Metabolism can be compared to an engine. An engine takes fuel and burns it to create power and heat. The power generated by the engine moves the vehicle. When we feel the hood of a car that has generated work, we find that some of the heat produced by the engine has warmed the hood.

Metabolism, like the engine of a car, takes fuel (energy from food or fat cells) and converts this energy into heat and power. We see the outward manifestation of this process in physical work, or movement of the human body. When we touch an individual who has exercised for a long time, they are warm to the touch.

Unlike the engine of a car, a real live human being is always generating heat. The amount of heat and energy expended by a human being is quite miraculous. Every single day, 24 hours a day, a human being, generates heat.

The fact that the human body does not destroy itself after a year or two of continuous work, but rather continues to work for some 60 to 80 years, pays tribute to the knowledge and wisdom that has been programmed into this wonderful part of the human body called metabolism.

Variable Speeds

Metabolism's speed is a variable phenomenon for human beings. Sometimes it is fast, other times it is slow. The amount of fuel consumed by an idling car engine is different from the amount of fuel consumed by that same engine as it accelerates from 0 to 60 mph. Likewise, metabolism uses less fuel (energy from food or fat cells) during sleep compared to the amount of fuel it uses to play a football game.

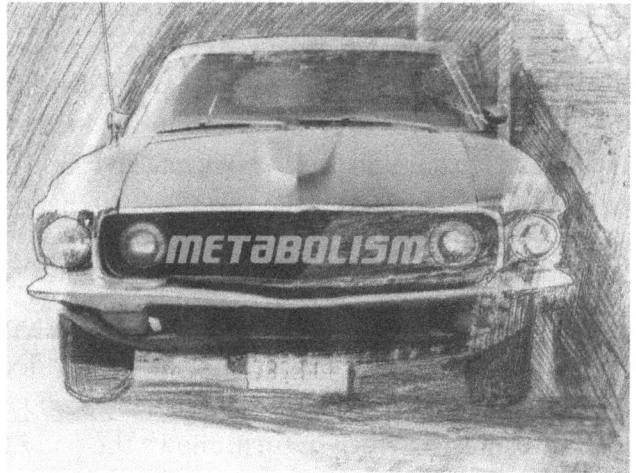

The resting metabolic rate, or idle speed for human beings is the amount of work done by metabolism when the body is awake, but at rest. Are some people's metabolic rate faster than others? Yes, and we will learn why as we progress through this book. The important thing to understand at this point in the investigation is this: Periods of time between waking up, and going to sleep, are periods of time where metabolism is constantly changing its rate of fuel consumption.

Of greatest interest, are periods of time between the football games and sleep, since these periods present variable speeds for metabolism. These speeds are dependent upon the combination and orientation of two variables, the Nourishment Triangle and the Physical Activity Triangle. One can adjust an engine to idle fast (burn more fuel), or slow (burn less fuel). Unfortunately, humans are not able to adjust their own metabolism speed manually, so in order to burn fat, we must use the variables to maximize metabolism's energy expenditure.

Is there an orientation of these variables (N-Triangle & PA-Triangle) that will maximize the amount of work done by metabolism in the course of the day, and thereby burn more food and fat cells? Yes, of the two orientations considered, one is very fuel efficient while the other one is not. If we compare metabolism to the engine of a car, what engine do we want? Would it be a small gas efficient engine, or a gas guzzling, 8-cylinder, muscle car from the 60's? In order to lose fat, we need metabolism to burn lots of fuel, like the engine of a muscle car!

The concept behind the Bases Loaded Plan represents the best orientation of the triangles, to boost metabolism consistently through the course of a day. To better understand why the Bases Loaded Concept is the best method, and as part of the analysis, we have to understand the dynamics between metabolism and the two triangles (variables) separately.

The reorientation of the N-Triangle and the PA-Triangle advocated by the Bases Loaded Program implies the notion that timing of food and physical exercise play a critical role in obtaining weight loss results. To understand why the metabolism reacts differently with the new orientation, we will create four models or experiments.

In the next chapter, we will first consider how food affects metabolism. We will look at how metabolism reacts to morning food with no daily exercise and we will look at how it reacts to evening food with no daily exercise. Thereafter, we will consider the relationship between metabolism and physical activity. We will look at how metabolism reacts to morning exercise with no daily food and we will look at how it reacts to evening exercise with no daily food. Before we look at these visual models that will help us understand the Bases Loaded concept in greater detail, let us pause and discuss the format that we will use to view the models. We will then review some of the material we have just learned in this section.

Model Format

Since metabolism is a phenomenon that occurs within the body, we will create models within the outline of an abstract human figure **(Figure 05)**.

As in previous models, the bottom of the rectangle represents the beginning of the day when the body wakes up. The top of the rectangle represents the end of the evening, when the body goes to sleep.

We will again use the dark and light triangles to represent food and physical activity respectively. We will use the medium shade to represent the inward engine "metabolism." This is an appropriate shade since "the medium" is a combination of light (physical activity), and dark (food).

The Metabolism Model Format

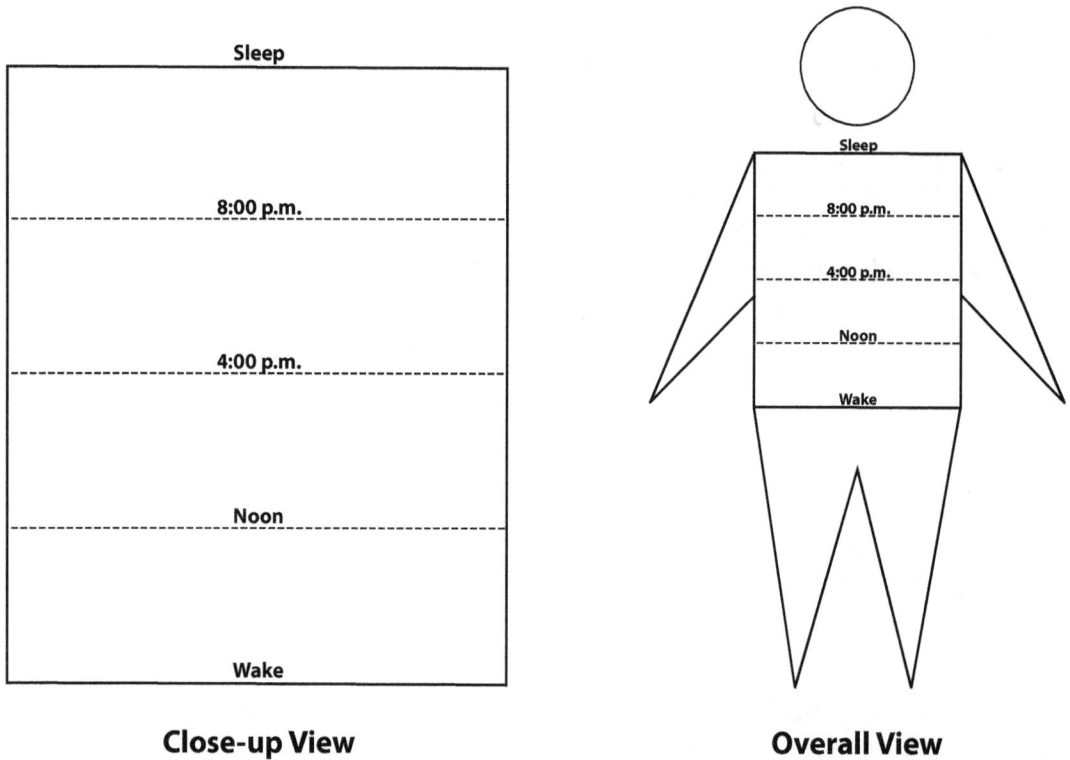

Close-up View

Sleep

8:00 p.m.

4:00 p.m.

Noon

Wake

Overall View

Sleep

8:00 p.m.

4:00 p.m.

Noon

Wake

Figure 05: Model Format - We will use a close-up view and an overall view to render visual representations of metabolism under varying conditions.

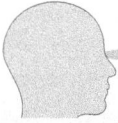

Check Your Understanding

1.   **True or false, the Bases Loaded concept advocates eating food late at night?**

   Answer: *False, the plan advocates eating during the day.*

2.   **True or false, the Bases Loaded concept advocates doing most physical activity in early and late evening hours?**

   Answer: *True, the plan advocates nightly physical activity.*

3.   **Which part, or system of the human body is responsible for transforming the food we eat into energy?**

   Answer: *Metabolism transforms food into energy.*

4.   **Is it true that a slow metabolism is genetic?**

   Answer: *False, metabolism is a variable phenomenon.*

5.   **According to the Bases Loaded Concept, what are the two primary variables, which affect metabolism's intensity at any one time?**

   Answer: *Food consumption and physical activity are the two variables that affect metabolism.*

How would our metabolism react if we sat at the computer all day and ate most of our food at night?

Metabolism Models

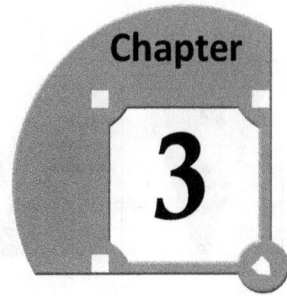

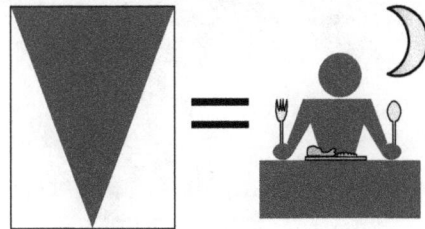

Metabolism Model #1: Night Food and No Physical Activity:

This first model shows the relationship between food and metabolism when we refrain from physical activity and eat at night.

We see from Metabolism Model #1 **(Figure 06)** the metabolism builds to a low intensity, proportional to the low food consumption in the early part of the day.

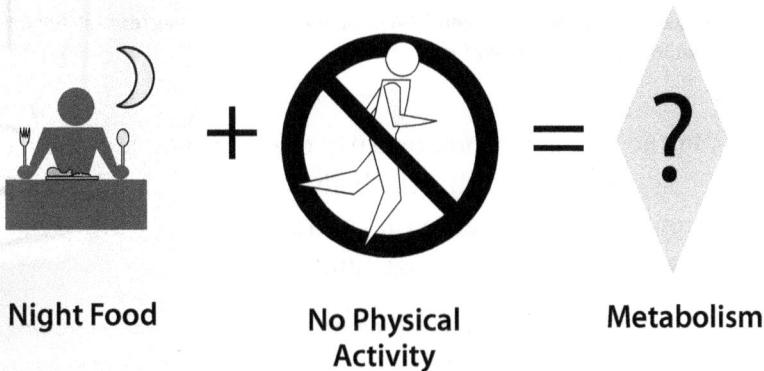

Night Food   **No Physical Activity**   **Metabolism**

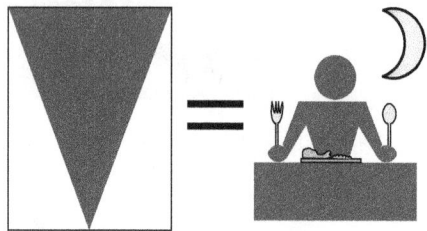

Metabolism Model #1

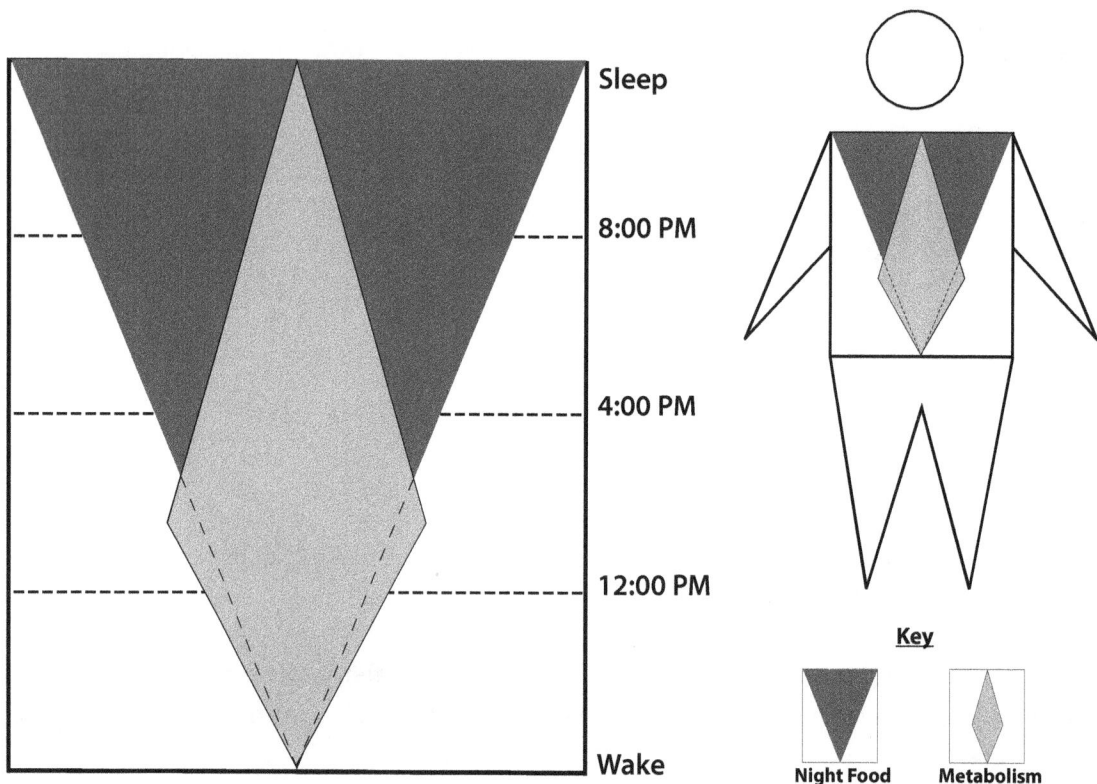

Figure 06: No Physical Activity & Night Food - Between 12-4 p.m., metabolism never reaches full intensity. From 4-8 p.m., metabolism slows down to prepare the body for sleep.

Look what happens in the late afternoon or early evening. The metabolism has already started to diminish in intensity, preparing the body for sleep. At night, instead of burning food, the metabolism chooses to conserve this extra energy for future use. By design, it diverts this extra fuel to its unlimited storage tanks (fat cells).

The trouble is the body seems to become more efficient at storing fat in the evening. As mentioned earlier this is in keeping with the body's internal clock, which slows metabolism starting in mid- to late afternoon-just as evolution was wired to do.[5]

Weight Loss Equation

In the model, we can subtract the medium shape of the Metabolism Diamond from the dark shape of the Nourishment Triangle to figure out the net amount of weight loss or weight gain. To help visualize this subtraction process, we have provided a visual entitled "Weight Gain/Loss Equation" **(Figure 07)**.

The best way to understand this equation is to think of the metabolism shape as a big eraser. As we overlap the triangle that represents food, we erase both the food triangle and the metabolism shape at the same rate. We erase them both until one of them cancels out. Graphically, this canceling process usually requires two steps. When the canceling process is complete, the shape with the most surface area will leave part of its shape intact. If the leftover shape is dark, then we have a model that represents weight gain. In other words, the metabolism output for the day was not able to erase or cancel out the amount of food consumed. The leftover food was thus converted to fat.

Metabolism Model #1 Weight Gain/Loss Equation

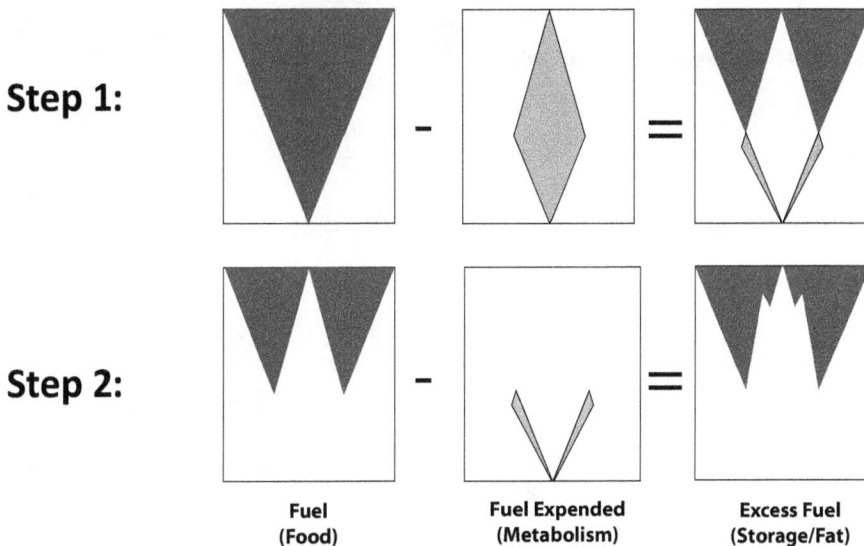

Step 1:

Step 2:

| Fuel (Food) | Fuel Expended (Metabolism) | Excess Fuel (Storage/Fat) |

Figure 07: Model #1 Weight Gain/Loss Equation - When we subtract metabolism from the amount of food consumed during the day, we see that Model #1, no physical activity and night food, represents weight gain.

On the other hand, if the leftover shape is medium shaded, then we have a model that represents weight loss. In other words, the metabolism output for the day was able to erase or cancel out the amount of food consumed. In addition, metabolism had to borrow energy from its storage units (fat cells) to meet the energy demands of the day.

From this equation **(Figure 07)**, we see that the net result of this model as indicated by the dark shaded shapes, represents weight gain. If we were to choose this model of very low activity and food consumed at night as a lifestyle, it is predictable that we would gain weight at a steady pace.

Observations #1

- **Metabolism has an internal clock which causes energy expenditure to slow down in the afternoon causing the body to store fat.**

- **Food eaten in the late afternoon and evening will be stored as fat.**

- **Model #1 represents weight gain.**

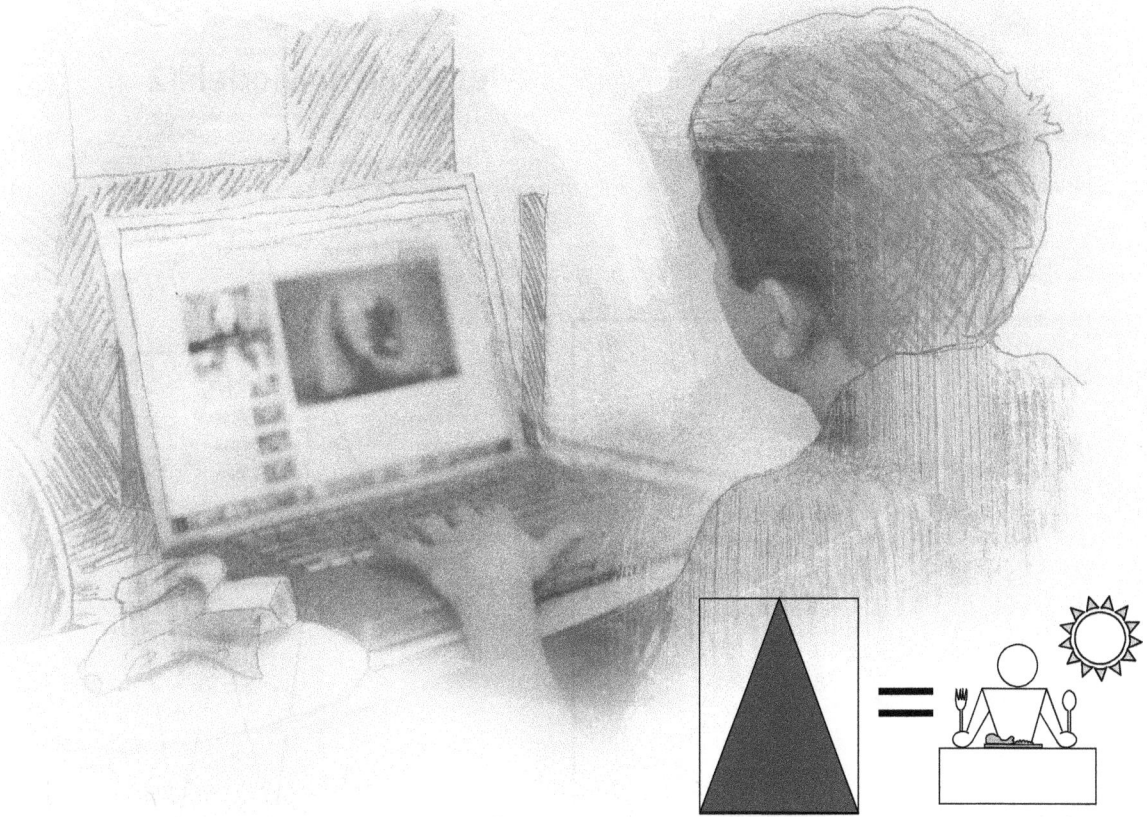

Metabolism Model #2: Morning Food and No Physical Activity

How would the metabolism react if we sat at the computer all day, ate the same amount of food as in the previous model, but ate most of the food in the early hours after waking?

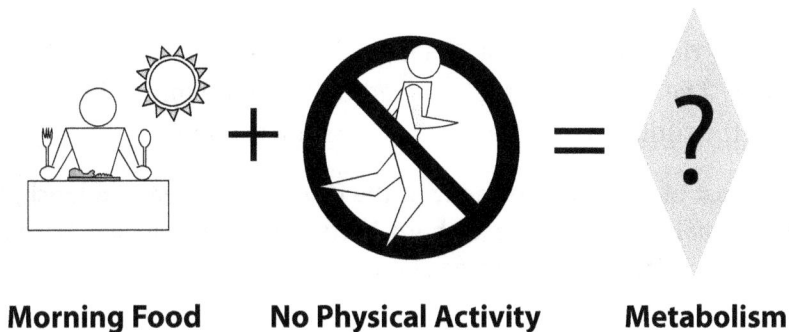

Morning Food   **No Physical Activity**   **Metabolism**

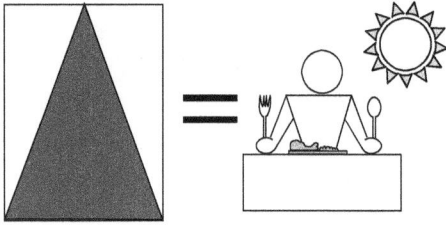

Metabolism Model #2

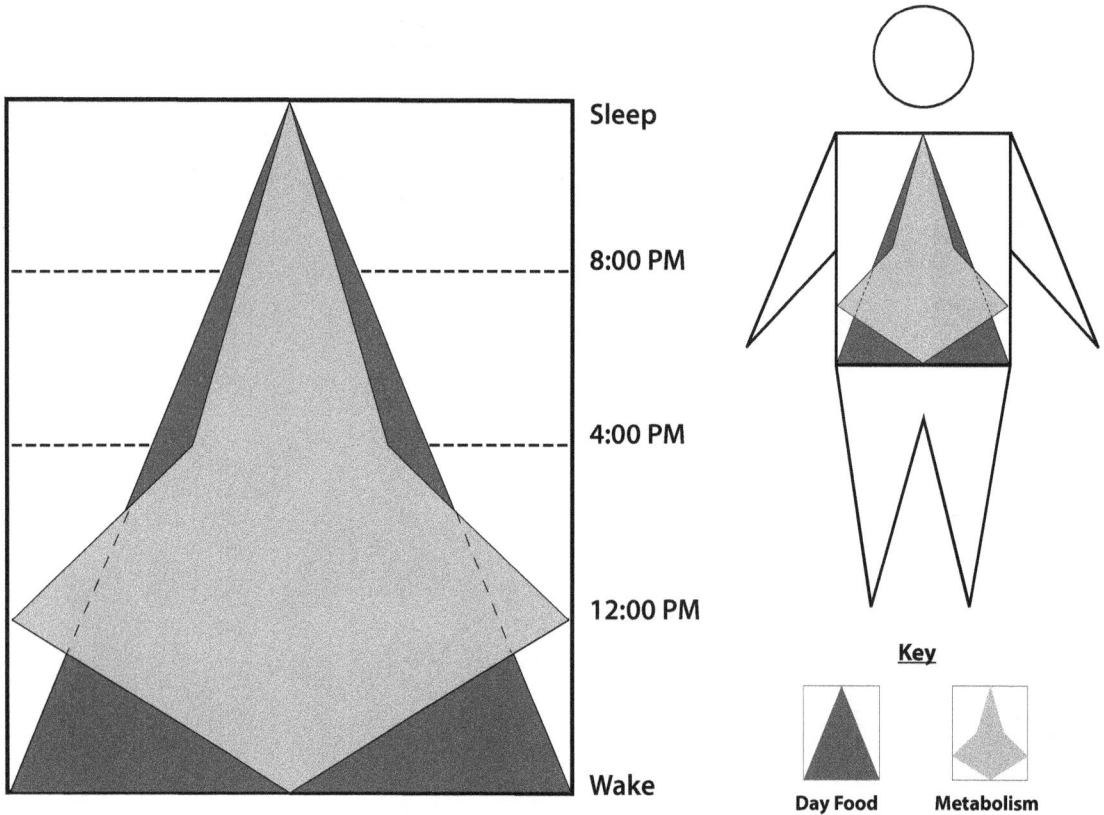

Sleep

8:00 PM

4:00 PM

12:00 PM

Wake

Key

Day Food   Metabolism

Figure 08: Morning Food & No Physical Activity- Metabolism burns energy intensely when food is consumed in the morning hours. Metabolism slows down in the evening hours to prepare the body for sleep.

By simply reversing the Nourishment Triangle, **(Figure 08)**, we find that something interesting happens. The amount of fuel burned by metabolism in this second model is greater. Evidently, the timing of food consumption is important.

Actually, if you get most of your calories early in the day-at breakfast and lunch, for example-you'll stoke your internal metabolic fire to burn hotter, according to Pat Harper, RD, MS, a spokesperson for the American Dietetic Association.[6]

Weight Gain/Loss Equation

As in the previous model, metabolism starts to diminish in intensity during the late afternoon. At day's end when we subtract the Metabolism Diamond from the Nourishment Triangle **(Figure 09)**, we find that metabolism is still unable to burn all of the food consumed during the day. The extra food that needs to be converted to fat is not as great as the amount we found in Metabolism Model #1, but it still represents a model of weight gain.

Metabolism Model #2 Weight Gain/Loss Equation

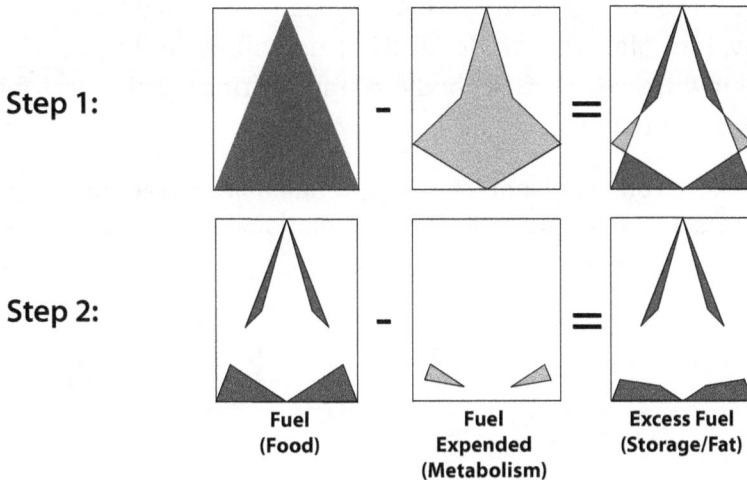

Step 1:

Step 2:

| Fuel
(Food) | Fuel
Expended
(Metabolism) | Excess Fuel
(Storage/Fat) |

Figure 09: Model #2 Weight Gain/Loss Equation - When we subtract metabolism from the amount of food consumed during the day, we see that Model #2, morning food with no physical activity, represents weight gain.

These two models teach us two highly significant things about metabolism and its relationship to food.

First: The metabolism will burn more food in the early waking hours of the day. Thus, all other things being equal (food quantity), timing of food consumption is important.

"In a University of Minnesota study in which all the participants followed a 2,000-calories-a-day diet, those who consumed most of their calories early in the day lost weight-2.3 pounds per week, on average-while those who ate later gained weight." [7]

Second: While the second model represents less weight gain when compared to model #1, it is still weight gain rather than weight loss. We need to cancel out the Nourishment Triangle, causing the body to dip into its energy storage tanks (burn fat cells), to furnish the daily energy requirements of the body. We thus need to incorporate the other variable, physical activity, into Metabolism Model #2. This will not only stop the body from becoming fatter, but it will also cause the body to start getting rid of excess fat. Like it or not, the human body needs to move.

Human-like creatures have existed on this planet for as long as four million years, and for roughly 99 percent of this time, they were hunters and gatherers." [8] **Evolutionarily, we were not designed to vegetate.** [9]

Observations #2

- **Metabolism has an internal clock. Food eaten in the early part of the day will cause metabolism to speed up.**

- **Metabolism slows down in late afternoon and early evening and prepares the body for sleep.**

- **Metabolism Model #2 represents less weight gain than Model #1.**

- **The body needs physical activity in order to prevent weight gain.**

Hypothetical Metabolism Model #3: Morning Workout and No Food

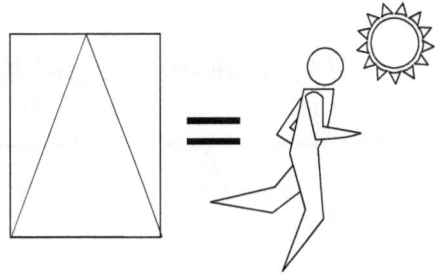

We have looked at the metabolism's relationship to food, let us now consider metabolism's relationship to physical activity. How would the metabolism react if we had a physical workout in the morning, and did not eat food the whole day? Let me preface my comments by stating, that the observations relating to the next two models derived from my own adult experiences.

Whenever we exercise or engage in physical activity, the inward engine must supply the necessary energy needs to the body. Therefore, the metabolism's intensity, is proportional to the intensity of the exercise.

"When you activate your energy with physical movement at regular intervals throughout the day, you sustain a consistently high metabolism.[10]

Logically, if we were to engage in physical activity all day long, the metabolism would expend energy all day long. What would happen, though, if we interrupted that physical activity with some rest, and did not allow ourselves to eat any food? That is what we are looking at in models #3 and #4, when we incorporate the variable of the Physical Activity Triangle and take away "food consumption" from the model.

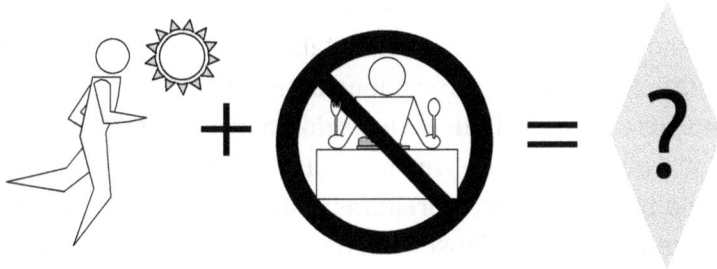

Morning Workout   **No Food**   **Metabolism**

Metabolism Model #3

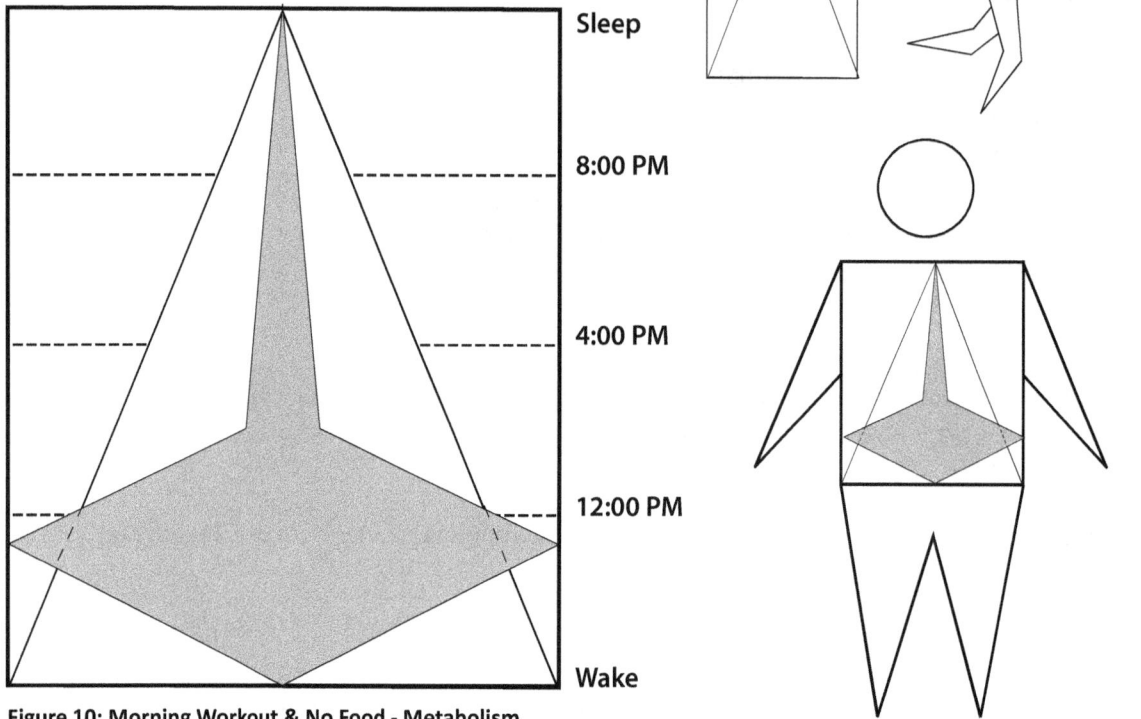

Figure 10: Morning Workout & No Food - Metabolism increases to maximum intensity during an early morning workout but slows down quickly, and continues to be slow throughout the afternoon and evening hours.

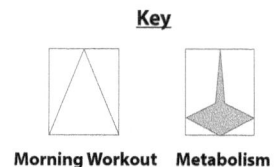

With the Physical Activity Triangle oriented so that a hard workout occurs in the morning, the intensity of metabolism maximizes early **(Figure 10)**. After this strenuous activity, when the body begins to relax, metabolism slows down drastically. This slowdown can be figured out using common sense. Those who have played a basketball game, or some other sport first thing in the morning before breakfast, have probably noticed that, after the game, they seem drained of energy. Those who have done this know that such a workout makes it hard to do the simplest of physical activities. This lack of energy is proof positive that the metabolism has slowed down.

Metabolism, as we explained earlier, is responsible for providing the energy needs of the body. The fact that the body feels no energy after a hard workout means that metabolism is limiting its allowance of energy expenditure. Put in other words, metabolism is conserving energy.

The solution to this problem is easy. What is it that we do to get energy back after a strenuous morning workout? We rest and then at some point we also eat some food.

We give the body some fuel. What happens if we do not eat some food? We feel tired all day. In other words, depriving the body of food, slows down metabolism.

Our "genetic programming" gives our bodies ability to control the production of enzymes, which in turn, control every aspect of our metabolism. Due to this fact, your body will "fight back" when you severely reduce food intake-it decreases the rate at which it burns fat.[11]

As indicated above, reducing food consumption also reduces fat burning. Physical work or exercise then reinforces this reaction of metabolism to slow down the rate at which it burns energy. Without the consumption of food, and having expended great energy in the early morning waking hours, the metabolism will slow down to conservation mode.

By afternoon the combination of a morning workout, lack of food and anticipation of sleep, keeps the metabolism in conservation mode. Once metabolism has arrived at this situation in the late afternoon, food will no longer jolt it out of its slow pace. The only thing that would cause the metabolism to speed up again is another workout. Such a workout would be extremely difficult for an adult and totally unrealistic for a child.

The total lack of energy a young person would feel after such a day's workout would send them to the couch early in the afternoon. There they would lay, able but unwilling to accomplish even the simplest of physical tasks.

Metabolism Model #3 Weight Gain/Loss Equation

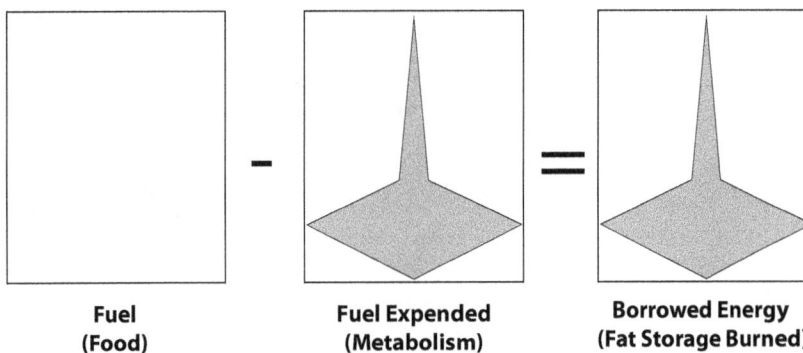

| Fuel (Food) | Fuel Expended (Metabolism) | Borrowed Energy (Fat Storage Burned) |

Figure 11: Model #3 Weight Gain/Loss Equation - When we subtract metabolism from the amount of food consumed during the day, we find that Model #3, morning workout and no food, represents weight loss.

Weight Gain/Loss Equation

A person would not need to worry about weight gain in the course of a day, following this model. The energy needs for this day, as indicated by the Weight Gain/Loss Equation, would be provided by fat cells.

In upcoming chapters, we will discuss how many fad diets follow strategies similar to models #3 and #4 to obtain quick weight loss. We will also discuss the reasons why such strategies eventually result in weight gain rather than weight loss.

Observations #3

- **Metabolism Is an energy regulator.**

- **Metabolism slows down to conserve energy.**

- **The combination of hard physical activity and lack of food in the early part of the day causes metabolism to drastically slow down.**

- **This model represents temporary weight loss.**
  Metabolism must burn fat storage to provide the body's energy needs.

Hypothetical Metabolism Model #4: Night Workout & No Food

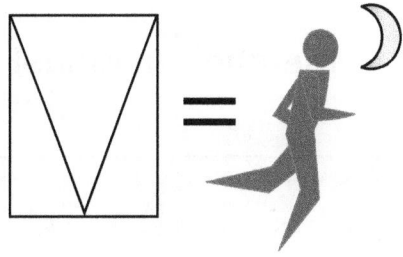

How would the metabolism react if, we did not eat food the whole day and had a restful morning, but a physically active evening ending with a workout?

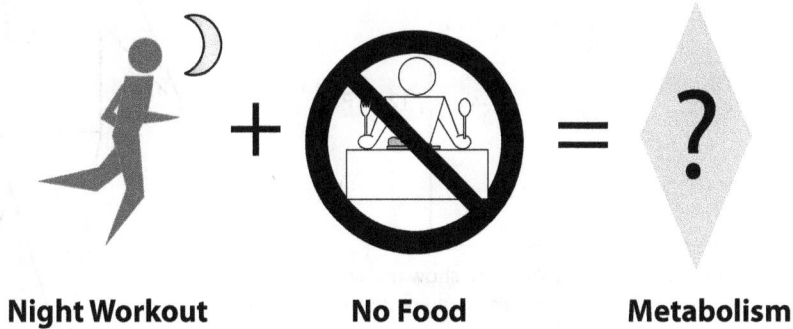

Night Workout   **No Food**   **Metabolism**

We see from the model **(Figure 12)** that, in the early morning hours, metabolism builds in intensity slowly, proportional to physical exertion. The metabolism never increases to full intensity during the morning hours. As the afternoon continues, metabolism starts to decrease in intensity, anticipating sleep.

In this model, the body engages in moderate physical activity, in the early evening, culminating in strenuous activity later in the night. Like the previous model, we see an increase in energy output by metabolism when physical activity is greatest. After a heavy workout, the big slowdown by metabolism conveniently occurs during sleep. To keep the models simple and consistent, we have not shown the shape of metabolism during sleeping hours. If we were to project the shape of metabolism in model #4, it would appear as a full diamond instead of a half diamond. In other words, the whole diamond that we see at the bottom of Model #3 **(Figure 10)**, would be reflected at the top of Model #4 **(Figure 12)**. The same workout, would thus produce the same reaction by metabolism, regardless of the time of day or night that the workout occurs.

Metabolism Model #4

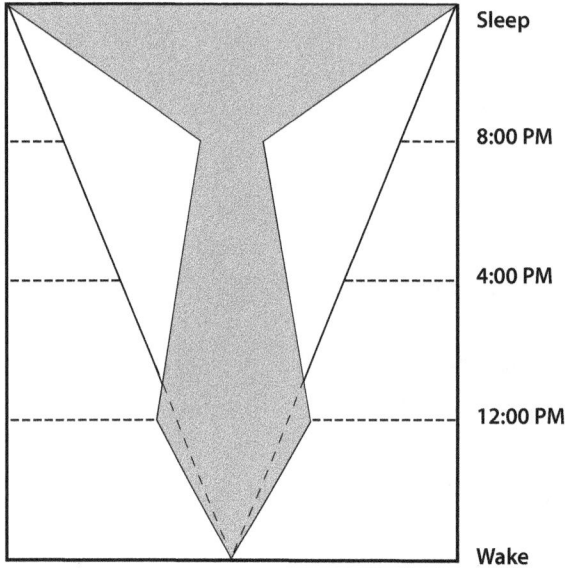

Sleep

8:00 PM

4:00 PM

12:00 PM

Wake

Note: Our model format does not allow us to show metabolism after sleep, but we can deduce that metabolism would reduce in intensity.

Figure 12: No Food and Night Workout - Comparing this model to our previous model, we find that delaying the workout till the end of the evening allows for greater energy during the day, to accomplish low level physical activities.

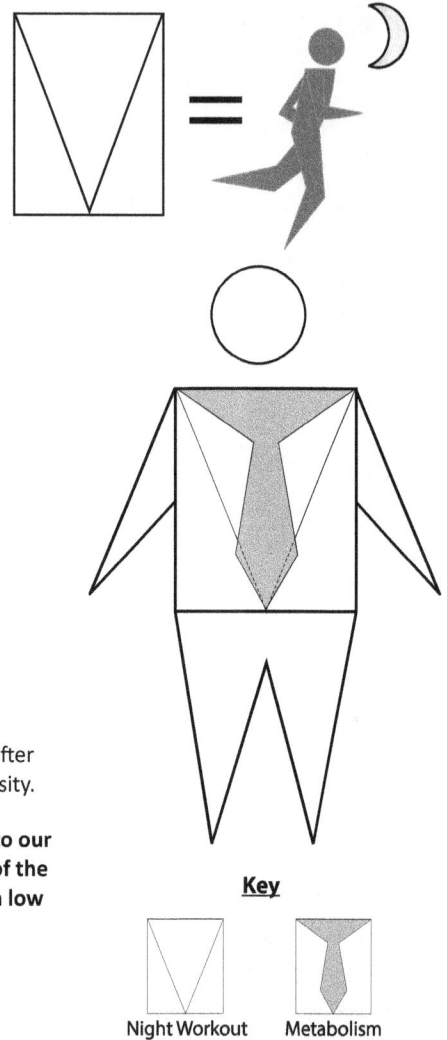

Key

Night Workout   Metabolism

Weight Gain/Loss Equation

Like the previous model where we looked at metabolism's relationship to physical work, the resultant of the Weight Gain/Loss Equation **(Figure 13)**, indicates a borrowing of energy from the fat reserves of the body.

Comparing this hypothetical model to the previous model, what do we find? If we were to add the medium shade needed to slow down metabolism to sleep mode, we would find that this model has slightly more medium shade of the two. Thus, this model represents the better scenario for energy consumption or fat loss.

Metabolism Model #4 Weight Gain/Loss Equation

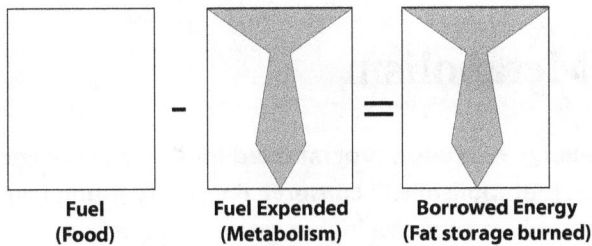

Fuel (Food) − **Fuel Expended** (Metabolism) = **Borrowed Energy** (Fat storage burned)

Figure 13: Model #4 Weight Gain/Loss Equation - When we subtract metabolism from the amount of food consumed during the day, we find that Model #4, night workout and no food, represents weight loss.

Observations #4

- **Metabolism is an energy regulator.**

- **Metabolism increases energy expenditure proportional to the work being done by the body.**

- **Delaying the workout until the end of the evening allows for a greater energy level during the whole day to accomplish low and moderate physical activities.**

- **This model represents slightly more temporary weight loss than Metabolism Model #3.**

- **Metabolism must burn fat storage to provide the body's energy needs.**

4 Model Synopsis

From these four models, we start to sense that metabolism is much more than a simple engine.

- **Metabolism is "an energy regulator."**

- **Metabolism's programming insures the survival of the human body.**

- **Metabolism acts as though human beings are still hunter/gatherers, interpreting food to be fuel or energy, and physical activity or exercise to be the body's search for food.**

We see from these models that metabolism works by some very predictable principles. Let us review these critical principles concerning metabolism.

8 Principles of Metabolism

1. Metabolism is an energy regulator, programmed for energy conservation. Metabolism is like the idle of a car. Metabolism will conserve energy by running at a low idle when the body is asleep. Metabolism runs at a higher rate when the body is awake.

2. Metabolism has an internal clock. It understands that the body needs rest in order to gather more food and energy. Therefore, the metabolism will slow down in the evening to prepare the body for sleep.

3. Early food consumption increases the metabolism's intensity dramatically. The metabolism interprets this early intake of energy to mean that the body has plenty of fuel and desires to find more fuel. Metabolism's programming allows for energy expenditure, when the body is in search of food. Believing that the body has the energy to spare, metabolism will allow the body to run at a faster pace so that it will successfully find more fuel.

4. Metabolism will not increase in intensity from the intake of food consumed in the hours before the body shuts down for sleep. Metabolism will continue to decrease in intensity as it prepares for sleep, and will send any extra fuel to energy storage units, or fat cells.

5. Metabolism starts the day in conservation mode. Without food consumption, strenuous exercise in the early hours of the day temporarily moves metabolism out of conservation mode.

6. Metabolism will increase proportional to the amount of work or exercise done by the body. Moderate exercise results in moderate energy expenditure by metabolism. Metabolism interprets exercise as the body's search for food.

7. Metabolism increases dramatically regardless of the time of day or night, when the body subjects itself to strenuous physical work or strenuous exercise. Metabolism interprets this expenditure of energy as a search for food.

8. Metabolism slows down dramatically after strenuous work or exercise when the body starts to relax if there is no early food consumption. Metabolism interprets this lack of available fuel, the high expenditure of energy, and the rest afterwards, as an unsuccessful search for food. Therefore, it slows down to conserve energy regardless of the time of day.

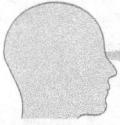

Check Your Understanding

1. **Does the metabolism run at a fixed rate, or does it run at variable speeds?**

    Answer: *Metabolism runs at variable speeds.*

2. **Does the metabolism naturally speed up, or slow down in the evening?**

    Answer: *Metabolism naturally slows down in the evening.*

3. **Without a workout, will the metabolism speed up, or slow down in the morning hours?**

    Answer: *It depends. Metabolism will speed up in the morning when the body receives sufficient food. If the body receives little to no food, metabolism will remain in conservation mode.*

4. **Is it true that food will always cause the metabolism to speed up?**

    Answer: *No, consuming food in the evening hours will not cause the metabolism to speed up.*

5. **What has the metabolism been programmed to believe about exercise?**

    Answer: *Metabolism interprets all physical activity as the body's search for food.*

6. **Describe the metabolism's internal clock.**

    Answer: *Metabolism understands that the body needs rest in order to obtain more energy. Therefore, the metabolism will slow down in the evening to prepare the body for sleep.*

7. **Is it true that physical exercise will always cause metabolism to speed up?**

    Answer: *Yes, Metabolism will increase in intensity proportional to the amount of work or exercise done by the body.*

8. **Why does metabolism slow down dramatically after a morning workout when the body starts to relax and there is no early food consumption?**

    Answer: *Metabolism interprets this lack of available fuel, the high expenditure of energy, and the rest afterwards, as an unsuccessful search for food. Therefore, it slows down to conserve energy regardless of the time of day.*

STRATEGY

GRAND SLAM

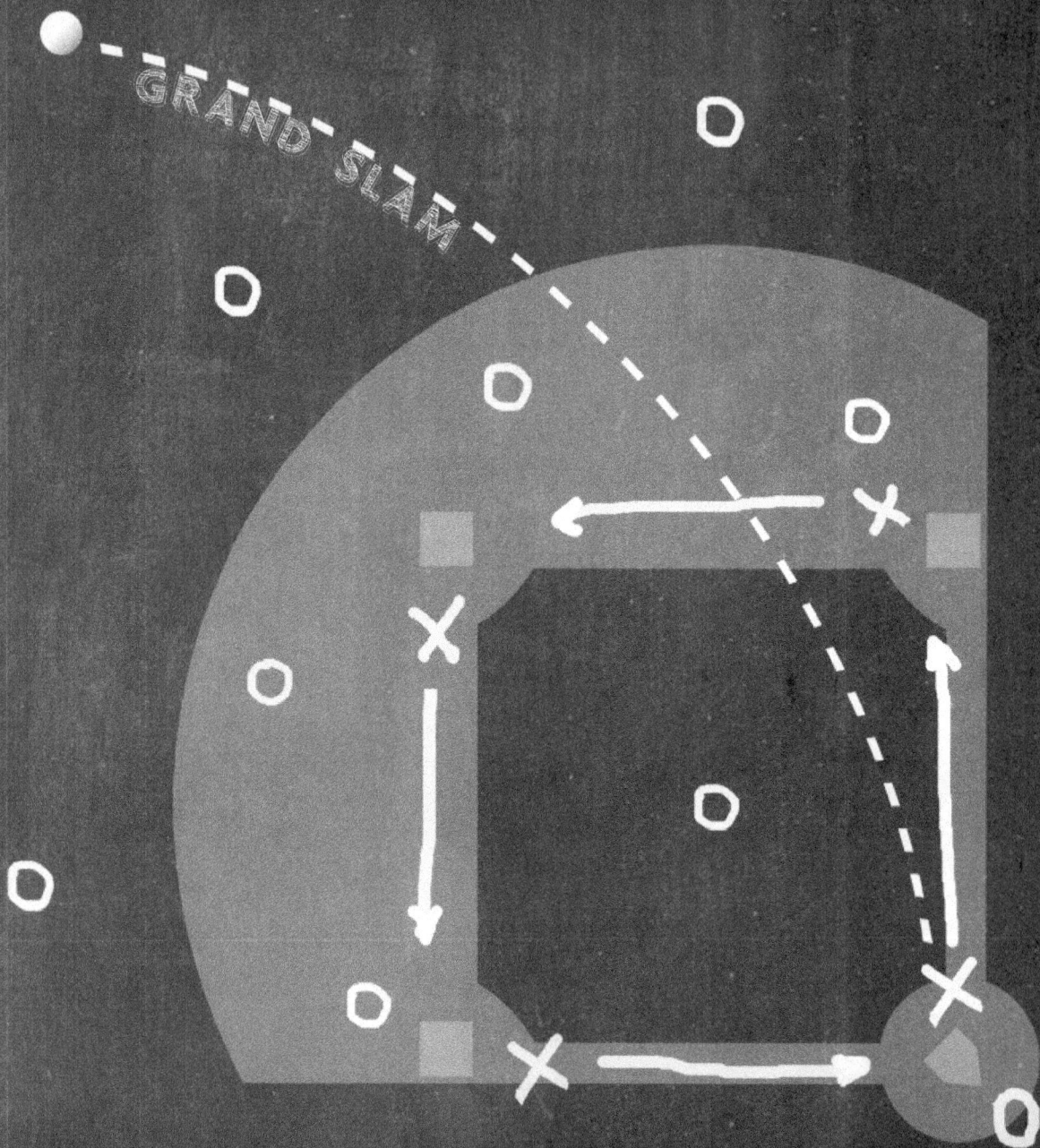

UNDERSTANDING THE PRINCIPLES THAT GOVERN
METABOLISM EMPOWERS US TO WORK WITH OUR
METABOLISM INSTEAD OF AGAINST IT.

The Bases Loaded Master Plan

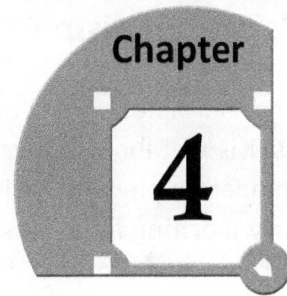

Composite Models

Now that we have a better understanding of the principles that govern metabolism, let us add up these observations into a visual comparison. This comparison contrasts the lifestyle of Joe before his program, to his lifestyle during his program.

The composite that represents Joe's lifestyle during his program is also a visual representation of "The Bases Loaded Program Master Plan." It represents a daily objective to work "with" metabolism instead of against it.

The master plan represents the best possible way to maximize the daily energy demands placed upon the metabolism. The metabolism must draw energy from the fat cells of the body to meet the energy demands of the day. It represents a safe, gradual method for young people to lose excess fat, and overcome childhood obesity!

In order to evaluate the Weight Gain/Loss Equation properly, we must visually eliminate the Physical Activity Triangle from these next two models. It is evident from the analysis that outward physical activity is deceptive. It is not the true indicator of weight loss. The Physical Activity Triangle is a mere shadow of the real work that is of note to us in these comparative composite studies.

The medium shade of the Metabolism Diamond is the true indicator of weight loss. It is the body's metabolism that determines how much fuel transforms into heat and energy. These next models thus retain the dark shade of the Nourishment Triangle, which is the symbol of daily food consumption. They also retain the medium shade of the Metabolism Diamond, which represents the burning of fuel by metabolism. The Nourishment Triangle and Metabolism Diamond thus represent "energy received" and "energy expended" respectively. With these two shades, we will be able to evaluate and compare the two respective lifestyles in terms of weight loss or weight gain. While the composite models visually strip away the light shaded Physical Activity Triangle, we will refer to the PA-Triangle in the key of the respective model description, **(Figures 14 and 16)**.

Joe's Metabolism Before Program

We see that before his program **(Figure 14)**, Joe receives very little food in the morning hours. His metabolism increases to moderate intensity in the morning hours due to low and moderate physical activities at school. The combination of physical activity and lack of early morning food causes metabolism's intensity to diminish in the early afternoon. By early evening, metabolism is operating in conservation mode, to prepare the body for sleep. Joe's food intake increases through early evening and into the night while his metabolism continues to operate in conservation mode.

Composite Model
(Close up View)

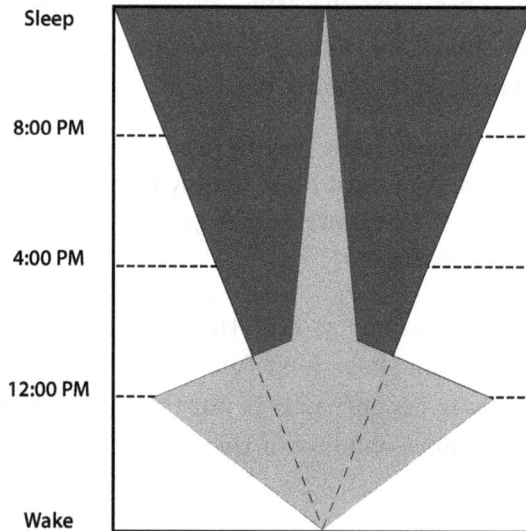

Key

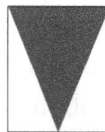

Night Food

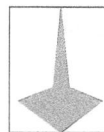

Metabolism
(Morning Physical Activity)

Figure 14: Joe's Metabolism Before Program - Lack of food consumption in the morning, with little physical activity in the evening, result in an overall, low intensity output by Joe's metabolism.

The Weight Gain/Loss Equation for this composite model **(Figure 15)** validates the gradual weight gain Joe experienced in his life prior to his program. The leftover dark shapes indicate an overall weight gain for the day.

Weight Gain/Loss Equation

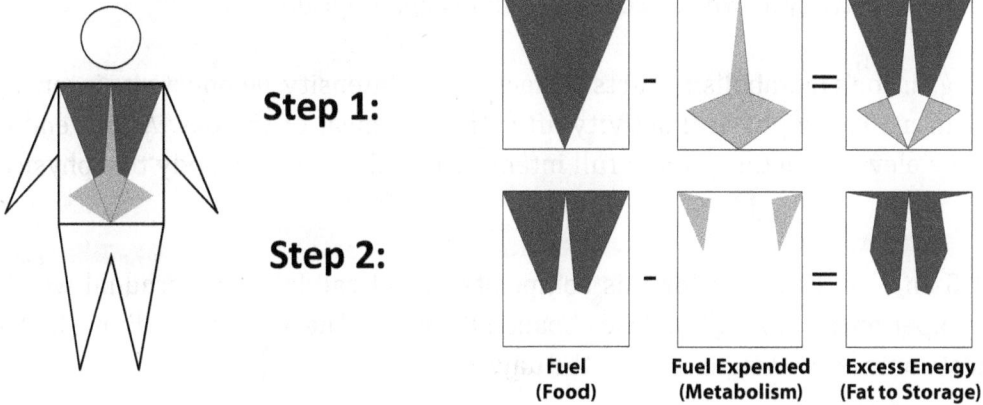

Step 1:

Step 2:

| Fuel (Food) | Fuel Expended (Metabolism) | Excess Energy (Fat to Storage) |

Figure 15: Composite Before Program, Weight Gain/Loss Equation - When we subtract metabolism from the amount of food consumed during the day, we see that this composite model, Joe's metabolism before program, represents weight gain.

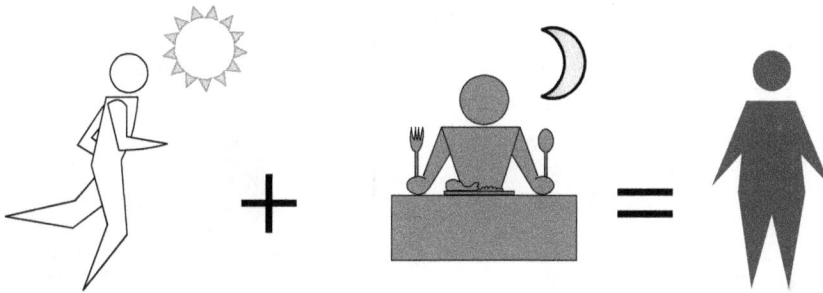

Joe's Metabolism During Program

The next visuals **(Figures 16 & 17)** exhibit the dynamics of metabolism in a typical day during Joe's program. Notice that this model combines the best two of the four models for food and physical activity that we studied earlier.

Eating most of his food in the morning causes Joe's metabolism to reach full intensity early in the day. Joe maintains high expenditure of energy during the day through low and moderate physical activity as well as continued food consumption.

In the evening, as Joe's metabolism starts to decrease in intensity, he boosts its intensity by engaging in moderate physical activity after the last meal of the day. At the end of the evening, he elevates metabolism to full intensity by subjecting his body to a physical workout.

The Weight Gain/Loss Equation for this composite model validates the gradual weight loss that Joe experienced during the Bases Loaded Program. The leftover medium shaded shapes indicate an overall weight loss for the day.

Composite Model
(Close up View)

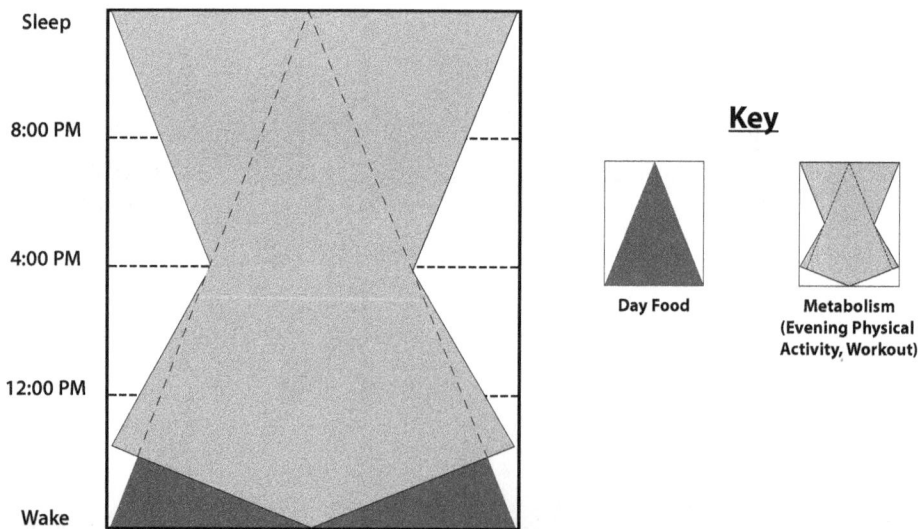

Figure 16: Joe's Metabolism During Program - Food consumption in the morning and afternoon, with evening physical activity and workout, result in an overall, intense output by metabolism.

These models are not quantitative, but we can use some simple math to obtain a rough estimate of what these shapes represent in terms of weight loss. On average, Joe lost about a half a pound of fat a week during the program. Near the end of the program, Joe exercised harder in his workouts and lost as much as a pound in one week. With this information, we can estimate that the leftover medium shaded shapes, represent a burning of between one to two grams of fat per day.

While one or two grams of fat loss per day does not seem like much, the effects of this slow but sure method over the course of a years time translates into 25 to 50 pounds of fat loss! Now that is impressive!

During Program
Weight Gain/Loss Equation

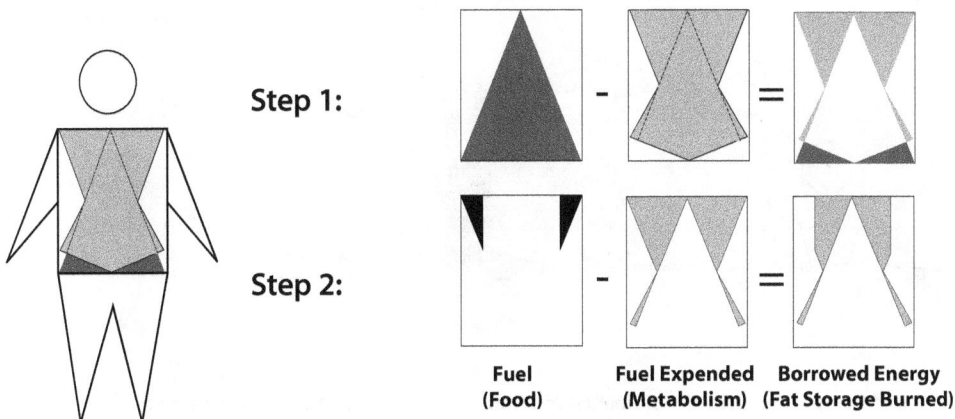

Step 1:

Step 2:

| Fuel (Food) | Fuel Expended (Metabolism) | Borrowed Energy (Fat Storage Burned) |

Figure 17: Composite During Program, Weight Gain/Loss Equation - When we subtract metabolism from the amount of food consumed during the day, we find that this composite model, Joe's metabolism during program, represents weight loss.

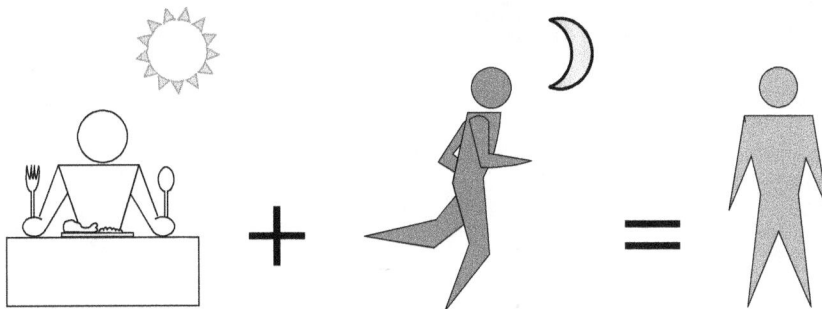

Simplified Models

Lifestyle <u>**BEFORE**</u> the Bases Loaded Program

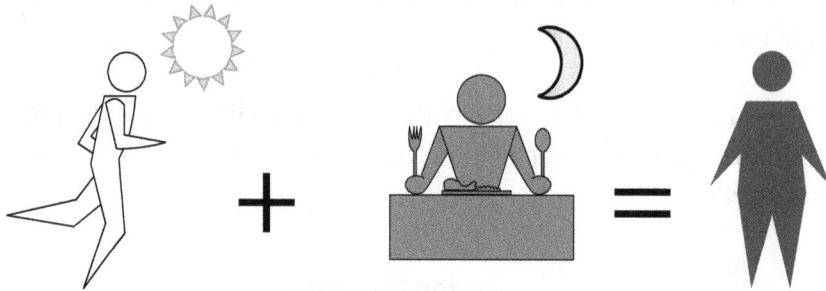

Lifestyle <u>**DURING**</u> the Bases Loaded Program

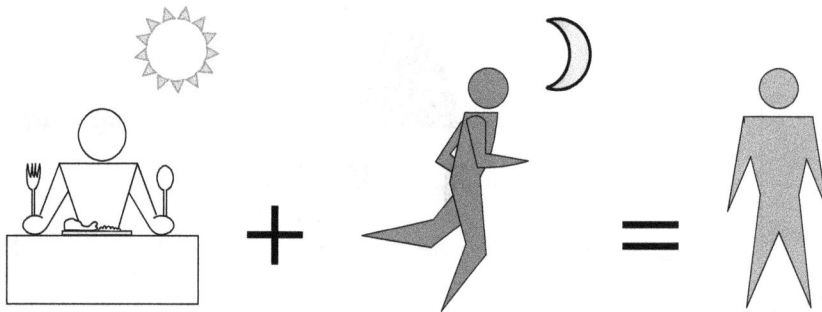

Figure 18: Simplified Composites - We can simplify our composites by thinking in terms of a mathematical equation. Even though the factors are equal in terms of quantity, we see that the orientation, or order that those factors are placed, yields different results.

Appearances can be Deceiving

Ever wonder why some people who exercise daily never seem to lose weight? Ever notice the "heavy set" weightlifter who is strong as an ox, but cannot get rid of his huge belly. I believe the next visual images **(Figure 19)**, help explain this paradox. Understanding the principles that govern metabolism, empowers us to work with the metabolism instead of against it.

Calorie counts are not important in the Bases Loaded Program. I honestly do not know how many calories compose different types of food items. Instead of channeling my mental energy into such knowledge, I concentrate on following correct principles and let my metabolism do the rest! If I eat nutritious food during the right time of the day, and combine that fuel intake with physical activity at night, I can have the peace of mind that I am not losing the battle against obesity! It sounds too good to be true, but it is true! This program gets "you" back in control of your body. It truly is a liberating feeling.

Before Bases Loaded   **During Bases Loaded**

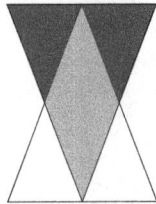

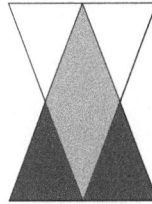

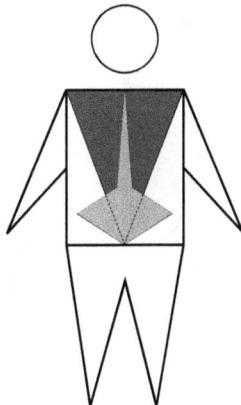

Inward Reality before Bases Loaded   **Inward Reality during Bases Loaded**

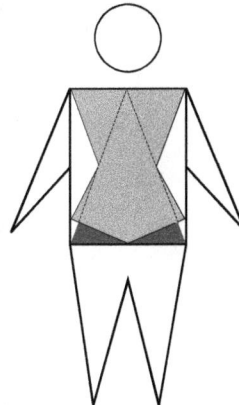

Figure 19: Appearances can be Deceiving - While the outward appearances of the two models shown above are very similar (same amount of food and physical activity), we see that the orientation of the two triangles within each model has a profound effect on the inward reality of metabolism.

Front View

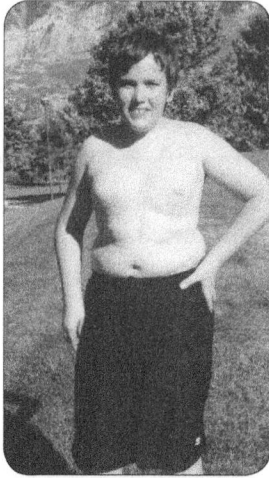 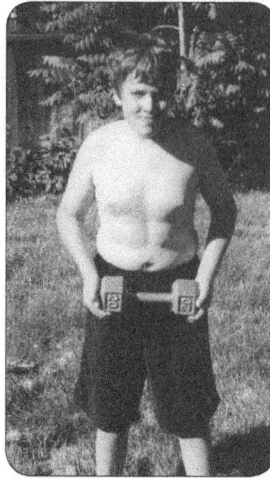 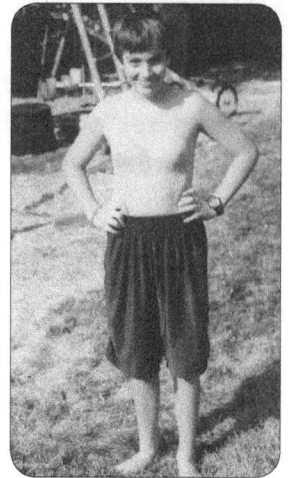

Back View

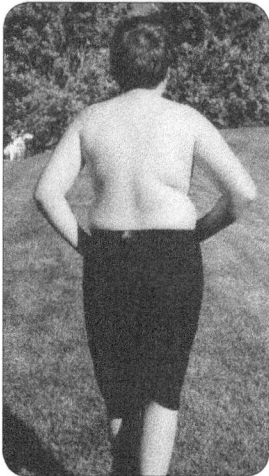 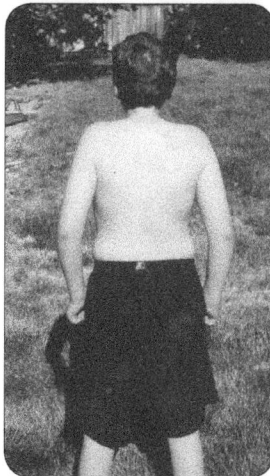 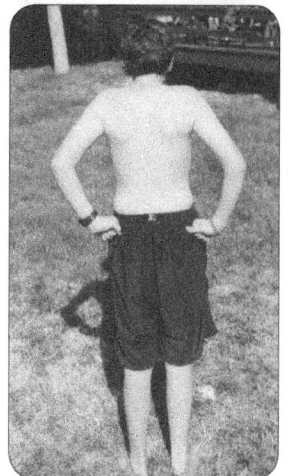

Side View

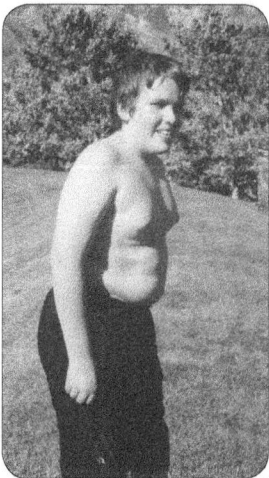 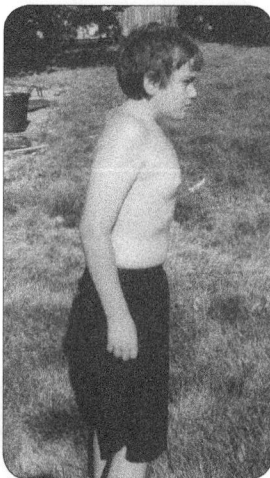 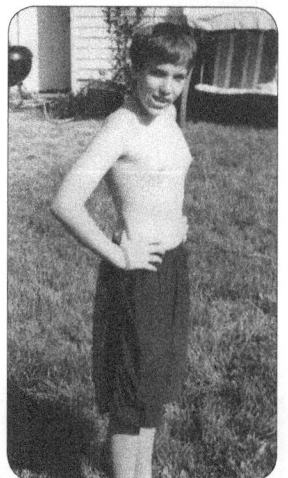

| Oct 1, 2005 | June 21, 2006 | Sept 9, 2006 |
| 143 lbs. | 123 lbs. (Lost 20 lbs.) | 108 lbs. (Lost 35 lbs.) |

Joe's Results

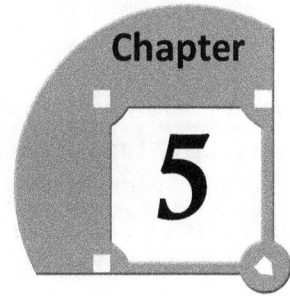

Joe began his program Oct. 1, 2005. That day he weighed 143 pounds. My wife and I sat down with him and together we all made a goal. Joe felt good about trying to lose 20 to 25 pounds. That would get Joe down to the weight that his pediatrician suggested. That goal meant that he would need to lose about two pounds a month or half a pound each week during the upcoming year.

Joe accomplished his goal of twenty pounds on June 21, 2006. When Joe lost 10 more pounds, my wife became worried. "Maybe he will lose too much weight!" So we looked at the growth charts that compare height for weight. We measured his height and found that he fell in the 75th percentile. The 75% for weight was 108 pounds. We all felt good that this was Joe's ideal weight. On September 4, 2006 Joe achieved his goal of 108 pounds. From start to finish Joe's program lasted eleven months and four days.

Like the flowers emerging to the sun and rain, it was the beginning of a new life for Joe and our family.

He Ain't Heavy, He's My Brother

Each picture below contains hand weights representing the weight loss Joe accomplished at the respective time of the picture. Joe had a tough time smiling holding the weights at the end of his program, so we enlisted the help of his brothers. Think about it, Joe was carrying almost 40 lbs of "extra weight" at the beginning of his program, 24 hours a day, 7 days a week. With the weight loss, it is easy to understand why Joe wears a natural smile on his face these days!

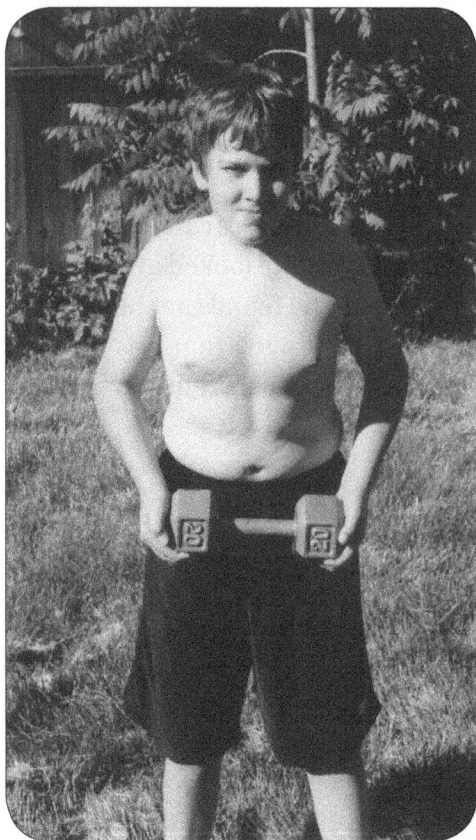

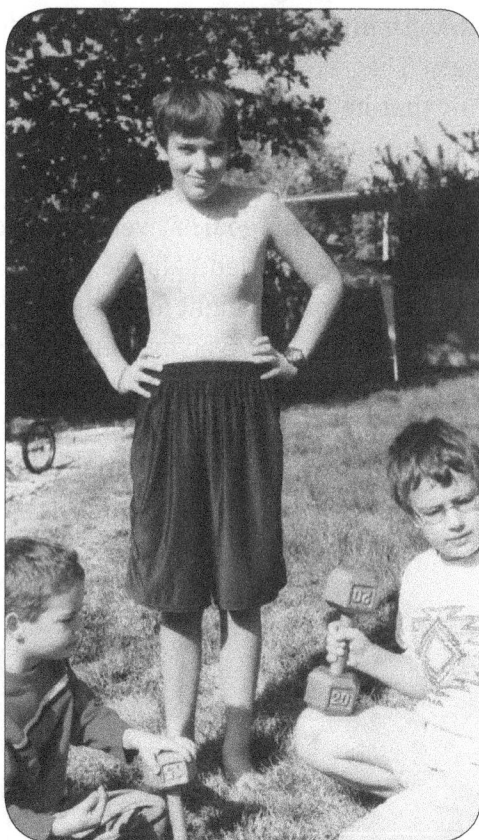

Joe's Reflections

Oct 1 2005—Beginning of Program

When I was younger I took pride in being heavier than my friends. I often boasted to my schoolmates saying, " I am heavier than you, so my numbers are bigger." I thought bigger was better. Now I see the irony of my thinking.

Before my program, I had trouble hiking with the other boy scouts. I had such a hard time that I thought my lack of energy was genetic. I guess deep down I knew that my weight had something to do with my inability to keep up with the others, but I was just rationalizing things to avoid the truth.

The first time I actually confronted my weight problem emotionally, was when my dad took those first photos, when I weighed 143 pounds. When he asked me to take off the shirt, I suddenly felt vulnerable and aware of my weight. I had shirtless photos taken of me at the beach or the pool, but this was different. The smile you see on my face was forced. Inside my heart, I felt horrible.

I guess you could say that those first pictures captured a low point in my life. I thought I was ugly that I couldn't do anything, or be good at anything. I didn't have many social skills, so I felt like a failure.

Many things started to change for me around the time I lost twenty pounds.

I was feeling a little thin. My confidence was starting to grow. My dad took pictures of me again, and we compared them to the photos that he took at the beginning of my program. My dad had hid the first photos from me, so when he pulled out the old photos and set them next to the photos where I lost 20 pounds I was shocked. I had no idea that I had lost so much weight! Looking back on the experience, I still had a long way to go, but this event had a huge impact on my life. Comparing the photos, and seeing the physical changes in my body got me excited. I started to believe that I could succeed at achieving the weight loss that I desired. The photos gave

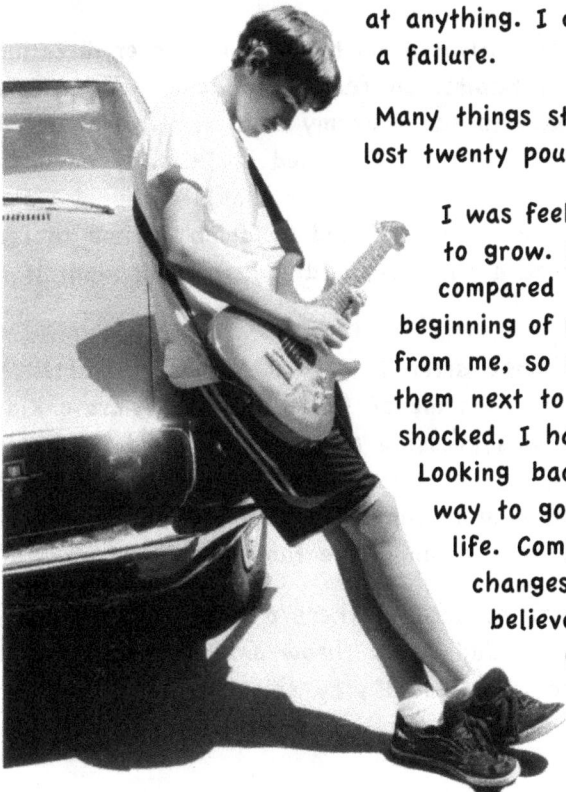

me physical proof that the hope and confidence that I felt were real. In particular, the photos helped me in my attitude towards workouts.

June 21, 2006—Lost 20 pounds

In the early stage of the program even the fun activities like riding a bike felt like work. Now I was finding that I had more endurance in activities like biking. I felt that my workouts were making a difference and so I started pushing myself out of my comfort zone.

I stopped focusing on the pain but looked at the satisfaction that I felt after doing a good workout. I started to realize that the pain of exercising was an important part of the whole experience and that life was more exciting or full if I experienced both the pain and joy. Life was definitely more exciting for me than the earlier times when I would sit around and watch TV while I snacked. I guess I knew that the workouts were getting me stronger. I was feeling more satisfaction in my life, and I am the type of person that loves satisfaction.

The new set of photos had an effect on my eating habits. I stopped cheating myself. In the early part of my program, I actually cheated and hid some Halloween candy under my bed and ate it without anyone knowing it. I realize now that the only person I was fooling was myself.

The photos showing the 20 pound weight loss motivated me to go in the other direction. I became very disciplined about my eating habits. In fact, my dad thought I was too disciplined. In looking back, I would have to say that my main motivation at this point was a motivation of fear. I was fearful that if I messed up once by having a dessert when the family went out to eat, or if we ate dinner too late that I would end up looking like the "old me" again. I guess it was kind of dumb for me to feel so paranoid, but I was starting to experience a new life, and I just didn't want it to slip away from me.

My relationship with my dad started to change after I lost 20 pounds. I started to see my dad as a mentor. Our relationship reminds me of the movie "The Karate Kid." At first, before I lost the weight, my dad was pressing me forward. I did not really like it, but I knew it was good for me. After I lost that first 20 pounds I still felt him pushing me forward, but I was now pushing in the same direction. Our friendship increased, and we started to joke around together and have fun.

I have many good memories of the program. My dad, brothers and I would go to the high school track in the summer evenings. My dad would throw a bucket of baseballs to each of us as we took our turn at bat. We would play sometimes until the sun went down.

The smiles that you see in the photos where I lost 35 pounds are not fake. I was very happy on the inside and outside. I had actually achieved my weight loss goals, and I felt like a new person! In many ways, I was a new person.

For the first time in my life, I felt that I was in charge of my body. I understood how to maintain a healthy weight, and the principles of my program were now a part of my life. This new power in my life carried over into other parts of my life. I felt more confidence in school, and in my social skills. I felt joy and hope for the future.

Sept. 9, 2006—Lost 35 Pounds

I can compare the progress in my program, to driving a car. When I weighed 143 pounds, I was at speed zero. At the time that I lost 20 pounds, I was accelerating to top speed. When I lost 35 pounds, I was just enjoying the cruise.

I felt confident, in control, and a part of the world around me. I felt connected to my family. My relationship with my younger brothers and sisters was never bad, but I can definitely see how my program has helped my relationship with them grow stronger. The same is true for my relationship with my parents. The sacrifices that I made during my program have helped me appreciate the sacrifices that my parents have made for me.

My program changed my life. It set me in a new way, a positive direction. I feel that I am still headed in that positive direction. After my program, I continued home school for two more years. I started going to a charter school in 9th grade. I feel that the discipline I acquired through my program helped me become a better student. Learning seemed to be smoother. I enjoyed learning new things such as guitar and computer graphics.

My program helped me gain integrity as a student. When I first started the program I was not honest with my parents in terms of my assignments. When asked "Did you finish that assignment," I would sometimes lie. Like hiding the candy under my bed, I came to realize that telling a lie doesn't solve a problem, it only makes things worse. When it comes to my assignments, I am completely honest with my parents now. They may get upset when I forget an assignment, but I know that they love me and are just looking out for my future.

My program has helped me get through some hard times. Sometimes I feel like the character Rocky in the movie "Rocky Balboa." I have learned to "take the punches and keep moving forward."

I feel that I have developed socially and spiritually. I feel peaceful inside. I believe this peace comes from seeing the bigger picture of life, and the potential I have to achieve possibilities that I never saw before my program. I now see myself as a person who has been given certain talents, and that it is important to develop these talents. In my case, it is music. I love playing guitar. I take pleasure in working hard at it.

The rules of my program have become principles that I use to help me live a satisfying life. I no longer have to be told when or how to exercise. I mainly just do fun things on my own, like going on bike rides. I take walks to break up my homework studies. I very rarely workout at the end of the evening like I did when I was on my program because I do not have a lot of fat on me now. I play hockey during the school year and workout daily in the summer break.

I do not have to be told what foods to eat or when not to eat. I just follow the principles that have become a part of me. I eat most of my food during the day and do not eat anything after dinner. I am not paranoid if dinner is a little late some evenings. On such occasions, I just eat a smaller amount so that I will wake up hungry the next morning.

In terms of food, I continue to eat "healthy" food and take my supplements. I have to prod my dad to make sure that there is plenty of fresh fruit in the house. I live my life according to correct principles and the principles take care of my weight.

Post Program—Present

Overall, my program has helped me direct my life in a positive direction, not just in terms of weight control, but in terms of my whole self.

I think you can sum up my program by something I achieved last summer. Before my program, hiking was probably one activity that I hated. I could never keep up with the other boys. Last summer I was one of a handful of Venture Scouts that hiked seven mountains in six days! Not only did I meet the challenge and accomplish the task, but I loved it! It was an intense and hard experience that required all my physical and inner strength. After conquering the last mountain and looking out over the beauty of the earth below, the thought came to me that I could never have accomplished such a task without the experience of my program.

The advice that I would give anyone struggling with weight problems is to understand your trials and problems. Come up with a workable plan using the principles you learn in this book and stick with your plan. Never give up! This program helped me, and it can also help you.

Before we begin part two and learn more important principles and details of the Bases Loaded Program, let us review the principles contained in part one of the book.

✔ Check Your Understanding

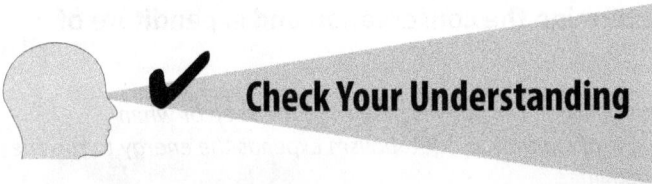

1. **In terms of weight loss, how much can one lose during a typical week, following the BL-Program?**

   Answer: *Following the BL-Program one should lose, on average, about half a pound a week, or two pounds a month.*

2. **Does the Bases Loaded Program require dieting?**

   Answer: *No, the Bases Loaded Program does not advocate dieting. The basic concept of the program is to reorient your eating habits. The bulk of daily food should be eaten within the first eight hours after one awakes in the morning.*

3. **True or false, the Bases Loaded Program requires a daily workout?**

   Answer: *True, the BL-Plan advocates a daily twenty-minute workout.*

4. **Should one workout in the morning or evening?**

   Answer: *Workouts should be at the end of the night, right before one goes to sleep. The program recommends that this workout occur six nights a week, with one rest day.*

5. **Is it true that skipping breakfast helps the metabolism to expend more energy during the day?**

   Answer: *No, just the opposite. Little to no breakfast causes the metabolism to decrease in intensity and conserve energy.*

6. **Does daily exercise in the morning guarantee that a person will lose weight?**

   Answer: *No, exercising in the morning often delays food consumption, which usually leads to food consumption in the evening hours. This in turn often leads to weight gain instead of weight loss.*

7. **Will eating the bulk of one's daily food in the morning, without daily exercise help one lose weight?**

   Answer: *No, eating in the morning is better than eating at night, but physical activity must be added to the daily routine in order to reduce the amount of excess fat a person has accumulated.*

8. **Are we "hardwired" to move like the ancient hunter/gatherers?**

   Answer: *Yes, the metabolism expends energy so that we may hunt and gather food.*

9. **What are the conditions that determine the conservation and expenditure of energy by metabolism?**

    Answer: *The metabolism conserves energy when the body is preparing for sleep or when metabolism believes the body is in danger of starvation. Metabolism expends the energy to run the human body and accomplish physical activities.*

10. **In starvation conditions with limited rations, would it be better for one's survival to eat rations first thing in the morning or late at night? Why?**

    Answer: *Under starvation conditions, it would be best to eat rationed food at night. Here, we find ourselves in a situation where we are trying to hold on to weight rather than lose weight. At night, the metabolism sends food to fat storage. Without food consumption in the morning, metabolism will keep the body running in conservation mode, thereby slowing the body's energy expenditure.*

Part Two:

The Working Model

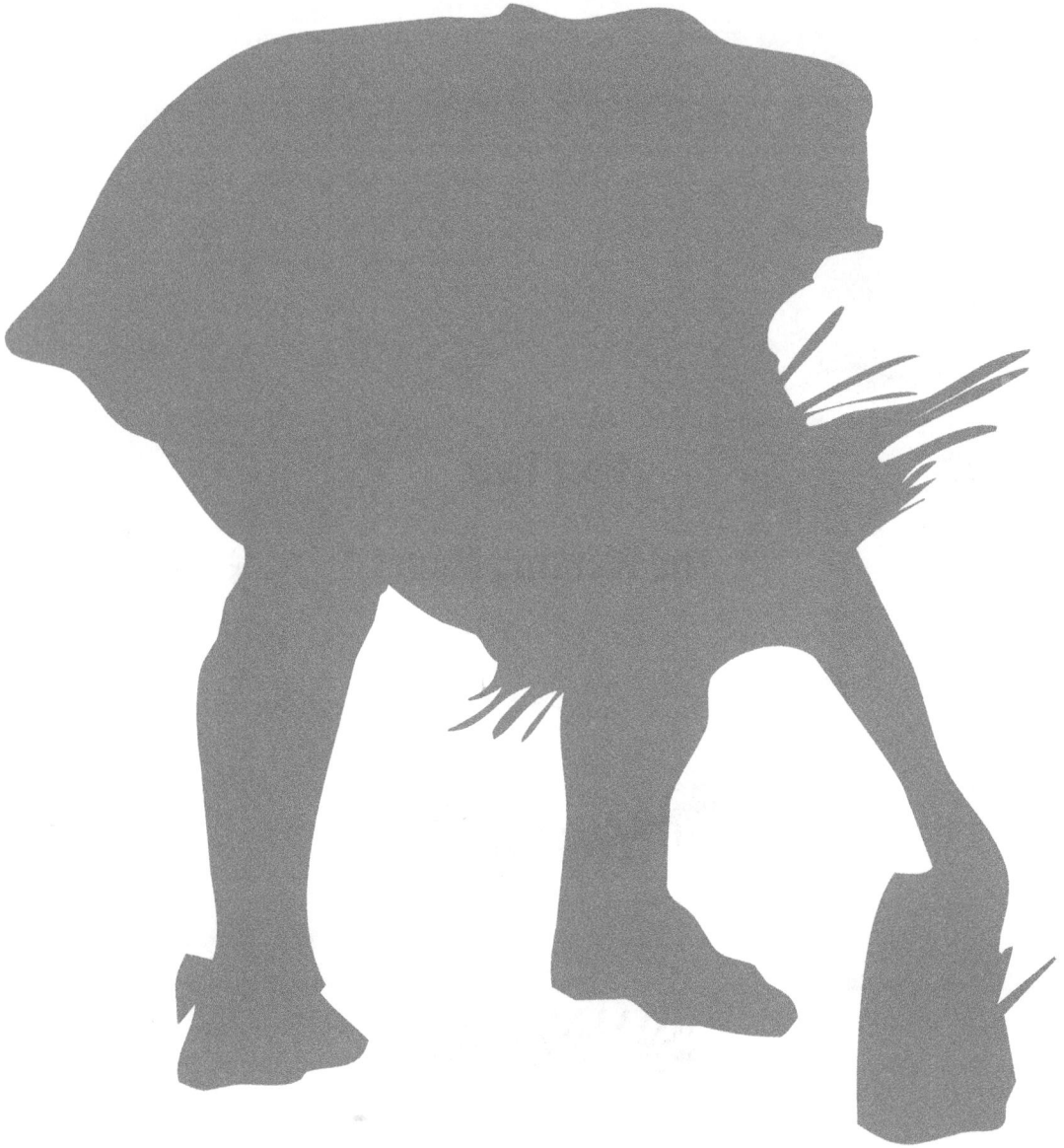

The closer we can come to mimicking the hunter/gatherer diet, or the nutrients they put into their body, the healthier we will become.

Food

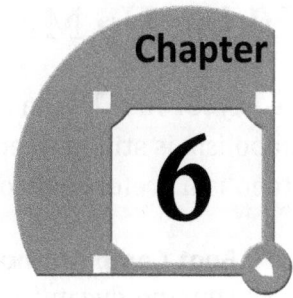

As we discussed in part one of this book, the metabolism believes that human beings are still hunter/gatherers. Can modern technology reprogram metabolism? No, therefore, we have to learn how to work with metabolism instead of fight it. In the next few chapters we will learn that working with metabolism means, sometimes we will want to mimic the hunter/gatherer ancestors, and in other cases, we will want to do the exact opposite of what the hunter/gatherers would do.

The metabolism manages energy received and expended by the human body. Half of what we need to know about the hunter/gatherers, therefore, revolves around the subject of "energy received," or food. The closer we can come to mimicking the hunter/gatherer diet, or the nutrients they put into their body, the healthier we will become.

"According to an expert in the field of evolutionary nutrition, Boyd Eaton, M. D., from Emory University: The principles of evolutionary adaptation suggest that if a dietary pattern is maintained within a lineage for nearly two million years, it must be optimal." [12]

"Remember those long-lost ancestors of ours I keep telling you about? The ones who were hunter/gatherers? Well, they all ate a very protein-rich diet. They didn't eat cookies and crackers and candy. And according to anthropologists, they were strong, had well formed bones, strong teeth, and they were rarely overly fat." [13]

Do not worry, this plan does not require exotic meals like buffalo burgers. Besides, the metabolism does not recognise food by its outward appearance. The composition of food includes proteins, carbohydrates, fat, vitamins, antioxidants, minerals, trace elements, fiber and water. These are some of the basic materials designed to help metabolism bring energy to the human body. There are plenty of meals that will deliver these materials to the body, and they will rival the taste of even the best buffalo burgers on the market.

Waking Up Mr. Metabolism

Here is your first lesson in learning to work with Mr. Metabolism. In the morning, your metabolism is still in sleep mode, and has to be woken up. There are four options, but Mr. Metabolism prefers only one of them.

a. **Boot Camp Method:** *"Rise and shine, get your butt out of bed Mr. Metab, we are running five miles, hitting the weight room, swimming a mile, all before 6:00 a.m. We have to get to work by* **7:00 a.m.** *What is taking you so long Mr. Metab, give me twenty push-ups right now!"*

b. **Saturday Morning Method:** *"Come on get up, I have two pages of chores written out on this yellow notepad and you will not have any fun today until all of them are checked off. There is no time for breakfast. I will fix you something when I see everything done to my satisfaction. Please start mowing the lawn."*

c. **Old College Roommate Method:** *"Good Morning, I have your usual breakfast ready for you, a cup of coffee and a cigarette. Hey, did you see in the paper, your team won again!"*

d. **Sweet Old Visiting Grandma Method:** *"Hi beautiful one, how well did you sleep last night? I am extremely glad. I made you just a little something to eat, a sourdough muffin with some reduced fat cream cheese melted on top because it is right out of the toaster. Would you like a little "all fruit" jam on top of that?"*

That is right; the correct method is (d), the "Sweet Old Visiting Grandma Method." The Boot Camp Method works for Marines and professional athletes. Not many of these types of professionals are fat. Most working people and children though have other things to do. If Mr. Metab could speak, his reaction to the Boot Camp Method would probably be something like this; "Fine, I'll do the five miles and all that other stuff, but unless you get me some food soon, I am going to take a nap, perhaps till tomorrow morning. I will let you deal with the rest of the day without my burning fire! Thank you, I hope you are happy with yourself, Sergeant Boot Camp!"

Old College Roommate method is convenient but takes a toll on the body. It is probably obvious that I had a college roommate, who, for breakfast, smoked a cigarette and drank coffee while reading the paper. He was one of my favorite roommates, but every morning he would wake up hacking and coughing. My other roommates and I would come home in the late afternoon and find him asleep.

Caffeine and nicotine are cheap counterfeits to the burning energy available from the metabolism. While they are convenient means to stimulate the body, they wear off quickly, asking the body for more of the same. Thus, these substances become habit forming, and end up replacing the nutrients a person might otherwise consume.

My old roommate's metabolism was probably saying, "Come on I want some real food, this stuff is fake! You keep this up, and you are going to be sorry. Your body parts are going to go on strike, and you will end up in the hospital. It will serve you right, and I do not mind because I hear they serve real food in the hospital, and anything is better than this fake stuff!"

Remember your mom writing that Saturday morning chore list? As a teenager, I vowed that I would never let my "adult" life be regulated by chores. Then I grew up and found that life had not changed much. The "Saturday Morning Method" is probably the most common method of waking up Mr. Metabolism. Perhaps it is conditioning or habit, but food first thing in the morning takes a truly low priority in the busy society we live. There seems to be too many important things to do and not enough time to do them.

The problem with this method of waking up metabolism is that it reverses the natural order of things. The metabolism transforms the food we receive into energy, which the body then uses to accomplish all of those necessary busy things we do. Doing the work before eating the bulk of one's daily food, leads to weight gain.

What does Mr. Metabolism say to us at the end of the day when we finally eat? "Now you send me this food? I needed this fuel hours ago. I have been working slow, waiting for this food! I am too tired to process it into energy right now. I am just going to send this to storage. You know I have an unlimited number of storage units available to me, and I am not afraid to use them!"

Believe it or not, one has to be like a sweet old grandmother if they want to please their metabolism first thing in the morning. A sourdough muffin with cream cheese is a snack that Joe eats occasionally. How would the metabolism react to such a kind, gentler approach? "Thanks, you must have been successful in hunting some saber-toothed tiger last night. Whatever that food was that I ate this morning, it sure was good. Excuse me a moment while I get my engines started; Grandma caught plenty of food for us today, and she is going out to catch more. We have work to do!"

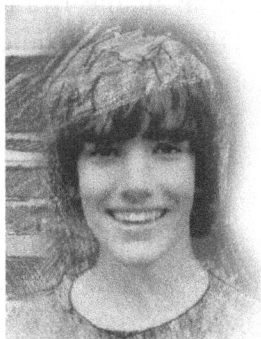

Like many people, before the program I wouldn't eat much breakfast. I would starve myself each morning until lunch. I would eat lunch and parts of my friends' lunch that they didn't want. After school, I would eat from the time I arrived home until it was almost time for bed.

In your program, you should have a short breakfast if possible, and a big breakfast to get your metabolism going. Then throughout the day, eat snacks. At around 5:00 p.m., have some dinner. Go for a walk around the block afterwards and do some fun things too. At 6:00 p.m., have a healthy dessert like fruit (not too much), before doing homework.

First Snack or Short Breakfast

Those that mow the lawn each week usually prime the engine by pushing a little bubble that sends a small amount of fuel to the carburetor. This small amount of fuel gets the engine going. Once the engine gets going, it automatically pumps more fuel to do the work of mowing the lawn.

Likewise, the first snack of the day primes the metabolism engine. Joe calls this first snack his "short breakfast." Below are some examples:

- **Sourdough muffin with low fat cream cheese, glass of orange juice, glass of water**

- **Two slices of 100% stone ground bread toasted, 100% natural peanut butter and all fruit jam, glass of water**

- **Homemade waffle, all fruit jam with banana slices, glass of orange juice, glass of water**

- **Apple with orange juice and peanuts, cup of water**

- **Small bowl of oatmeal with apple slices, Agave syrup, 1% milk, glass of water**

- **Toast with buttery spread enriched with omega-3 and peanut butter, banana, glass of water**

- **Baked sweet potato, glass of orange juice, cup of water.**

The short breakfast is a time to relax and wake up, read the paper or simply meditate. Make something that is enjoyable to eat. Let it be short and nutritious. It is important to have a glass of water in the morning. Be sure to drink enough water during the course of the day. Water is an essential element needed by metabolism and the digestive tract, to do the many jobs that they do. Prime your metabolism and get excited for the day. It is going to be a fabulous day!

Breakfast

Breakfast should be as large as your child wants it to be. Do not be concerned at this point of the investigation about the obvious dilemma of how to switch your child to eating a bigger breakfast. We will offer a suggestion concerning this matter in the "Getting Started" chapter.

Here are some examples of breakfast, Joe's way:

- **Two slices of cracked wheat sourdough bread toasted and buttered with a spread enriched with omega-3, two eggs enriched with omega-3 sunny-side up, a glass of orange juice, and a glass of water constitutes Joe's favorite breakfast.**

After Joe dips his toast, he likes to put ketchup and cayenne peppers on his egg whites. Some fruit rounds off the meal.

- **Breakfast #2: Ham and cheese omelet using two omega-3 eggs, one slice of lean ham, mozzarella or cottage cheese, with a little cheddar cheese mixed in, two slices of sourdough bread with omega-3 spread, 100% fruit jam, a glass of orange juice, a glass of water, and fruit**

- **Breakfast #3: Two homemade waffles with buttery omega-3 spread and 100% fruit jam, peaches cut up and put on top or the side, low fat yogurt, Agave syrup on top, a glass of orange juice, and a glass of water**

- **Breakfast #4: Big bowl of hot oatmeal with cut-up apples mixed in, top with a little Agave syrup and 1% milk, two slices of 100% stone-ground bread with omega-3 buttery spread and peanut butter, a glass of orange juice, and a glass of water.**

The size of the breakfast will vary according to the size of the person eating it. The rule of thumb for breakfast is simple, "Eat until you are satisfied." Enjoy every bite. Food is a good thing, not a guilty thing.

I Do Not Like Breakfast as Much as I Like Dinner

There are some, who do not like breakfast food as much as they like the foods associated with dinner. They are probably saying; "Where are the meat and potatoes?" "You want me to cut down on my favorite foods, the ones I eat at dinner and eat more of that mushy food that I ate as a baby?"

Spoken like a true hunter/gatherer! Remember, the hunter/gatherers did not have the luxury of the breakfast foods available to us now. The solution to this dilemma is easy, switch meals. Eat dinner for breakfast and breakfast for dinner. Those that enjoy meat and potatoes more than toast and eggs can switch meals. Heat up some of last night's leftovers in the microwave while other family members eat their eggs and toast.

Have the types of wholesome foods that are most enjoyable during the early part of the day. Have those wholesome foods that are enjoyable in small amounts as the last food of the day.

Timing Of Food

Once a person has eaten some food within the first hour of waking, how long should they wait before they eat some more food? To answer that question let us remember the new orientation of the BL-Nourishment Triangle. In terms of timing, the BL-Nourishment Triangle advocates getting most daily food within the first eight hours after waking from sleep. There is great flexibility in how we accomplish this task. Some people will prefer to eat a large breakfast followed by hourly healthy snacks till dinner. Other people will prefer to eat several small meals through the day. This food then is the base portion of the triangle. The top part of the Bases Loaded Nourishment Triangle, the point of the triangle, represents dinner and the last food of the day. As the tapering of the triangle suggests, we want to taper down the amount of food we consume at the end of the day.

Last Food

The last food of the evening should be consumed at least 12 hours before the first food of the next day. Thus, if we eat the first food of the day at 7:00 a.m., the last food of the evening should be eaten no later than 7:00 p.m.

The last food of the evening should also be consumed at least 3-4 hours before we go to bed. There are two reasons for this short abstinence from food. First, it is the design of the Bases Loaded Plan to keep metabolism running strong right up until the time we go to bed. As discussed earlier, food late in the evening translates into fat production and weight gain. Second, the BL-Plan calls for a 20-minute workout at the end of the evening. We want food to be fully digested by the time we have this last workout.

One of the great aspects of the BL-Plan is the wonderful feeling of freedom it provides. As one follows correct principles, they will find that the relationship they have with food will take on a new dynamic. No longer will "food" control them, but they will be the one in control. Food will take its proper role in their life. It will not only provide energy to perform daily work or study, but it will also be a source of enjoyment and pleasure.

Snacks:

Here are some examples of snacks that Joe enjoys.

- **An apple**
- **A banana**
- **An orange**
- **Cut up watermelon and honeydew melon**
- **100% whole grain crackers with peanut butter, orange juice**
- **A handful of mixed nuts**
- **Three pieces of string cheese**
- **100% whole grain crackers with low fat cream cheese, orange juice**
- **A peanut butter and jelly sandwich, orange juice**
- **Turkey or ham with cheese and mayonnaise sandwich, orange juice**
- **Bean or avocado dip with corn chips**
- **Carrots, celery, raw broccoli, with low fat sour cream dip**
- **Small portion of leftover healthy dessert, such as whole wheat banana bread or carrot cake**
- **Protein bar and orange juice**
- **Plain low fat yogurt with Agave syrup and/or blended berries.**

Principles to remember about snacks are as follows:

- **A snack is about a handful of food.**

- **It is perfectly fine, even preferable to have a few different snacks together. The larger principle, that we should eat food combinations, applies here.**

- **Like all the food we put into the body, snacks should be healthy.**

- **Snacks are frequent. The longest time between snacks is one hour. The shortest time between snacks is a half hour.**

- **Snacks should be easy to access. In my home, we lay out all the snacks on the kitchen table after breakfast is over. My family will munch on these snacks until dinner.**

Ideas for Packing Lunch

Perhaps your child eats a healthy hot lunch at school. Perhaps they bring their own lunch. Why not do both?

Here are some ideas for those who make lunch for children that attend school.

Use lots of sandwich bags and divide your food into "handful" portions or snacks. Wrap each half of the sandwich in its own sandwich bag. Encourage your teenager to eat these snacks between classes, as well as at lunch. Your pre-teen child may not have many opportunities to snack. They can eat many of the packed snacks for lunch. They can save the rest of the snacks for after school. Eating these snacks between school and dinner works well within the BL-Plan. Later snacks will reduce the tendency your child might have to overeat at dinner.

Ideas to Prevent Overeating at Dinner

Meals, unlike most snacks, are usually warm or hot. The digestive system likes to be pampered with the "Sweet Old Grandma Method."

The amount of food eaten at dinner should be modest, much less than the amount of food eaten at breakfast or lunch. Metabolism has worked all day long and wants to slow down. The danger with dinner is its tendency to tempt us to overeat. The digestive system sends a signal to the brain, "Oh, this food is so warm and good, keep eating!" Here are a few things that we can do to avoid overeating at dinner:

- While preparing dinner, have a snack. This little trick is easy to remember in my home. In order to eat dinner, we have to clear the table of all the snacks. Naturally, we nibble at these snacks while we carry the food back to the refrigerator.

- Limit your dinner to one plate of food.

- Drink plenty of liquids at dinner. It is okay to have seconds of orange juice or water.

- Incorporate low fat soups into your dinner. Soup satisfies that digestive yearning for something warm and comforting, especially in cold climates. A bowl of hot soup takes time to eat and allows dinner to be a social event. As with liquids, it is okay to have "seconds" as long as your soup is low fat.

- Put some cut-up fruit on the table for dinner. Cut-up oranges, grapes, or melons are extremely refreshing, especially during the warm months of the year. Having fruit on the table also curbs the desire to reach for seconds. Reach for some cut up oranges instead of potatoes. Having something naturally sweet at the end of a meal seems to round out the meal and gives one that "satisfied" feeling.

- Shortly after dinner, go for a walk. My family makes this a daily activity during the summer months. Walks allow us to gauge the amount of food we should be eating at dinner. If we have overeaten at dinner, a walk will seem impossible. A walk after a dinner extends the working limits of metabolism. It sends the message to metabolism that the work of the day is not yet done, and the body is not yet ready to go to sleep.

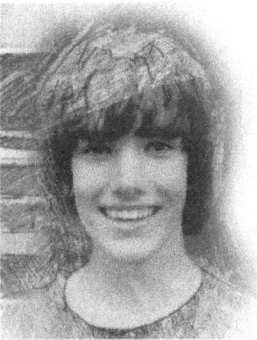

Instead of serving us lunch, my dad would set the table with a bunch of fruit, and foods that give you protein (peanut-butter for instance), veggies that kids like to eat (carrots, celery), and usually a dip of some sort. Kids like to eat this stuff and this stuff has 99.99% less junk than junk food! Do not make your kid's life like the Marine Corps, where you sternly growl at them and say, "Do not eat that," or "Stop eating so much!" This will affect the relationship you have with your child.

When it comes to snacks and food, the hardest part of the program for me was getting off the junk food. I guess my body was used to junk. I was used to getting sugar highs and maintaining that sugar high through the evening. Once I decided to be serious about the program and stop hiding candy under the bed, my body adjusted to a diet that had little junk in it.

Compare Energy Levels

Let us revisit the last visuals and look at them in terms of energy level. As before, the dark shade represents food. The medium shade represents metabolism, but also represents the energy level one feels throughout the day. Notice the difference. By feeding the metabolism early, we can count on more energy throughout the day. Notice the small amount of medium shade in the afternoon of the "Before Bases Loaded" visual. Ever yawn or feel sleepy about 3 p.m? Compare this to the afternoon portion of the BL-Plan. By eating one's food before early afternoon, and mixing in some low and moderate physical activity, we create a new scenario. The metabolism will build a huge fire that will continue throughout the morning and into the afternoon.

Bases Loaded advocates the eating of nutritious food. The next chapter will concentrate on nutrition principles. As we diligently incorporate these principles into family life, food will become a source of health, satisfaction, and pleasure.

Before Bases Loaded Program   **During Before Bases Loaded Program**

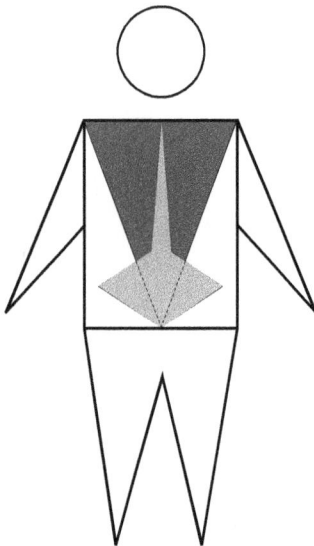

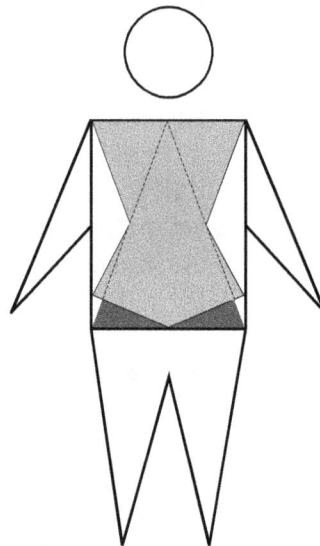

Figure 20: Comparing Energy Levels - The medium shade not only represents metabolism, it also represents energy levels. Comparing the two, we find that Joe's energy level was much higher while following the BL-Plan.

✔ Check Your Understanding

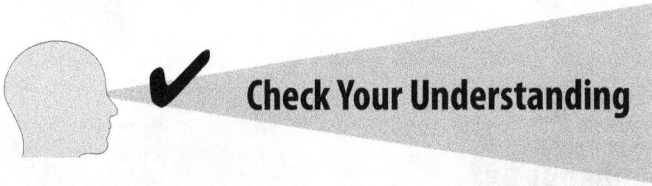

1. **Which method is metabolism's preferred method of waking up in the morning; Boot Camp, Saturday Morning, Old College Roommate, or Sweet Old Visiting Grandma Method?**

    Answer: *Metabolism prefers the Sweet Old Grandma Method.*

2. **When should the first food of the day be eaten?**

    Answer: *Within the first hour after waking have a short breakfast.*

3. **When should we eat?**

    Answer: *We should eat the bulk of daily food within the first eight hours of the day after we awake.*

4. **If one has their first food of the day at 7:00 a.m., when should they finish eating the last food of the day?**

    Answer: *At 7:00 p.m., have your last food.*

5. **What is the rule one should follow when eating breakfast?**

    Answer: *"Eat until you are satisfied," is the rule one should follow.*

6. **Does one have to eat breakfast food in the morning?**

    Answer: *No, one can eat any type of wholesome food in the morning.*

7. **How much food constitutes a snack?**

    Answer: *A snack is about a handful of food.*

8. **Is it okay to snack shortly before dinner?**

    Answer: *Yes, a timely snack helps reduce the tendency to overeat at dinner.*

Much of America's obesity epidemic can be traced back to a lack of understanding of these principles of nutrition.

Principles of Nutrition

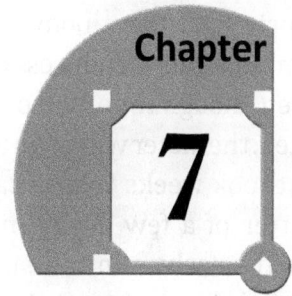

Chapter

7

Principle One: Eat a Variety of Healthy Food

There is a food that contains all the vitamins, minerals, proteins, carbohydrates, fiber, and trace elements one needs to get through the day. It is light but filling. It is mildly sweet and delicious to the taste. Though it contains fat, it is not fattening. It is the one perfect food. Unfortunately, no one ever bothered to jot down the recipe for "Manna from Heaven." If there were a perfect food, life would be easier. At the same time, according to the biblical account, even a perfect food like manna got boring to some people over time.

By design, food should be eaten in combinations. Food combinations are like the colors of the rainbow. An art professor once taught me that there is no such thing as a "beautiful color." A particular color appears beautiful because of the colors around it. So it is with food. There are few things more appealing than the taste of pink grapefruit after a breakfast of toast and eggs. Take the toast and eggs away and eat grapefruit all day for weeks on end, and at my house, the kids would come home to find large grapefruit-sized holes in the kitchen and dining room windows!

If most children are like Joe, they tend to gravitate towards carbohydrates rather than proteins and vegetables. Meats and green leafy vegetables were important to the hunter/gatherer ancestors, and they are an important part of building strong healthy bodies today. For Joe, incorporating principle #1, getting a variety of healthy foods, meant getting more protein, good fat, and vegetables into his diet.

"The fact is, our bodies work much better with a balance of carbohydrates and protein. You see, not only is protein essential for building healthy muscles and maintaining a strong immune system but it helps stabilize insulin levels as well." [14]

Diets that advocate or gravitate towards the eating of one particular food, while eliminating other foods, are boring. They also deprive the body of important nutrients. Interestingly, boring diets often cause the dieter to gain weight in the long-term. Here is how that happens.

Depriving the body of varied food combinations produces cravings. Cravings, given enough time, will overpower the dieter. Often, the dieter will go on a food binge. Pounds that took weeks to lose can be regained in a matter of a few days. Unknowingly, dieters put themselves into a situation where they are fighting against their own metabolism.

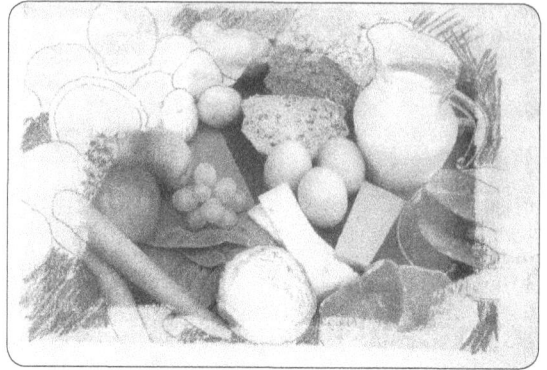

"If you starve your body of certain nutrients the next time you introduce it, your body will store it, which is what the body does in a time of famine." [15]

When the dieter gains the weight back, they feel guilty. They then resolve to be more disciplined in following the diet. So begins a very unhealthy cycle of diet and food binging. If the dieter is not careful, such habits could develop into serious problems, such as anorexia or bulimia.

Bases Loaded advocates a better way. Instead of creating a war where the human body fights against the human spirit, let us create a healthy marriage where spirit and body work together.

By eating a variety of healthy food, we will, in essence, create manna. Healthy food combinations will eliminate cravings. Instead of the body shouting, "I need some meat and potatoes!" at the top of its inner voice, and your spirit responding, "Be quiet and eat the grapefruit," we will have an inner conversation that goes something like this. "Honey dear, lover of my body, spirit of mine, put some of those potatoes and meat on the plate, will you baby?" "Anything for you, lover. What is that beautiful one? Of course, I will not forget the steamed vegetables."

The BL-Plan replaces the marital discord of "cravings" with the marital bliss of "hunger," and the satisfying of that hunger. There is a big difference between cravings and being hungry. Cravings, as discussed earlier, are indicative of an unhealthy situation. Being hungry is a natural phenomenon that we should feel when we wake up in the morning. It is simply the prelude to an extremely enjoyable meal.

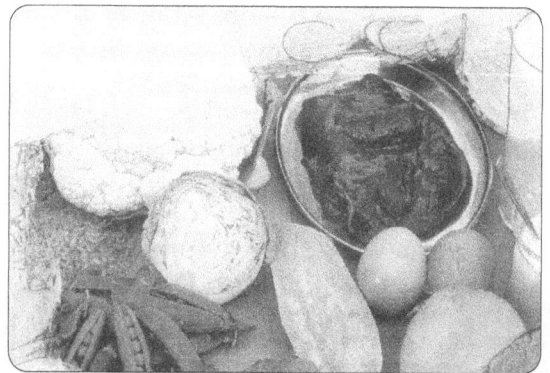

Principle Two: Avoid Junk Food

Junk food is like any other food in certain respects. Eaten over a long period at the exclusion of other foods, a junk food diet, will produce unhealthy results. Since junk food is primarily sugar, refined carbohydrates, bad fats, or a combination of these, they compound the health risks. The body is deprived of essential nutrients and taxed with unhealthy weight gain.

I have not heard of anyone who has woken up on New Years Day and said, "I am going to start a junk food diet this year!" If junk food diets are not a matter of preference, why do they just seem to happen?

The answer is simple; sugar and fat taste great! A deeper question to ponder might be, "Why is it that human beings of every culture love the taste of sugar and fat?" I believe the answer goes back to the old miser Mr. Metabolism.

There is evidence to suggest that these foods are addicting. I also believe the desire for fats and sweets to be instinctual. These foods taste good to all human beings because we are all programmed for survival. Metabolism views sugars and fats as quick and stored energy, important commodities to ensure the survival of the species.

This situation worked for the good of the hunter/gatherers. They would come across a berry patch, or a honeycomb once in awhile. They would eat and fill up with sweetness, but it was sweetness filled with fiber.

The composition of fats were also different. The fats that hunter/gatherers ate came from wild game that fed on wild plants, and so the fat content was different from the trans fat and highly saturated fat of junk food.

Not only has the composition of energy food changed, but the availability has changed, as well. We can now fill up with junk food each and every day, to metabolism's content.

"I call modern America the nation of the overfed and undernourished...Underfed on nutrients that help sustain life. And overfed on junk that takes life away." [16]

While Mr. Metabolism may be attracted to a junk food diet, the rest of the body starts to rebel. Like any other diet that excludes food combinations, a junk food diet will cause cravings. Along with these cravings, a diet high in sugar causes blood sugar to increase dramatically after eating, and then plummet. The combination of cravings and unstable blood sugar cause the junk food dieter to be perpetually hungry and tired. How do junk food dieters solve this low energy problem? They eat more junk food!

Junk Food Diet Cycle

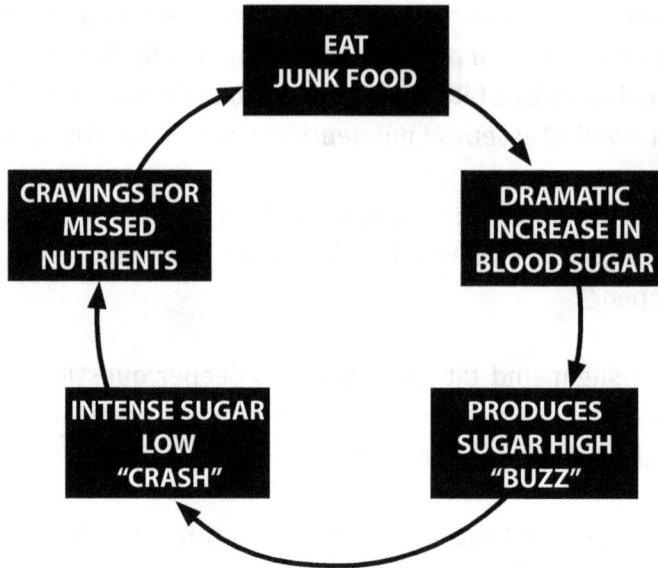

```
                    ┌─────────────┐
                    │    EAT      │
                    │  JUNK FOOD  │
                    └─────────────┘
      ┌──────────────┐          ┌──────────────┐
      │ CRAVINGS FOR │          │  DRAMATIC    │
      │   MISSED     │          │ INCREASE IN  │
      │  NUTRIENTS   │          │ BLOOD SUGAR  │
      └──────────────┘          └──────────────┘
      ┌──────────────┐          ┌──────────────┐
      │ INTENSE SUGAR│          │  PRODUCES    │
      │    LOW       │          │ SUGAR HIGH   │
      │  "CRASH"     │          │   "BUZZ"     │
      └──────────────┘          └──────────────┘
```

A junk food diet, like a binge diet, creates an unhealthy cycle. Instead of a cycle that completes itself weekly or monthly this type of cycle completes itself several times a day.

Breaking a junk food diet is challenging, but not impossible. If one eats most of their food at home, the solution is simple. Replace all the junk food with a healthy variety of food. When one gets hungry and reaches for potato chips, they have magically turned into carrots! Even children will eat healthy food when the food is convenient.

Eating your food outside the home requires a little planning. That money that is in your wallet for junk food needs to be spent on healthy food that can be made into snacks. Make some snacks before leaving the house. Stick them in your backpack along with a bottle of orange juice. Be sure not to replenish your wallet with money. Put enough in there to call home, but not enough to buy a bunch of doughnuts.

The BL-Plan calls for 98% healthy food and allows 2% for junk food. We will allow an occasional doughnut when shopping with your kind visiting grandma. Seriously, the key to avoiding a junk food diet is to be wiser than Mr. Metabolism. Remember, Mr. Metabolism is a miser when it comes to energy. He will try to get his host to eat as much high-energy food as possible by appealing to the taste buds. The next principle will teach how to be wiser than Mr. Metabolism when it comes to energy food.

Principle Three: Replace Quick Release Energy Food with Slow Release Energy Food

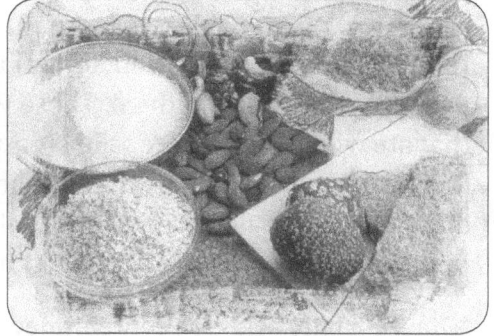

Junk food lacks nature's most magical ingredient, fiber. Fiber can be thought of as nature's packing material. As stated earlier, the metabolism interprets sugars and fat as quick energy, or potential energy to be stored.

Imagine in your mind, a conveyor belt delivering a bunch of energy molecules to your stomach. The conveyor belt keeps delivering them until your stomach feels full or sick. Now, imagine this same conveyor belt delivering the same energy molecules, but this time they are packaged in a fibrous material that has to be unwrapped.

The conveyor belt has to slow down because of this unwrapping process. The fibrous wrapping material fills up the stomach like a living room gets filled up with wrapping paper during a birthday party. When the stomach feels full, and we count the amount of energy molecules received into the stomach, they are significantly less than the batch without the packing material.

Fiber keeps the body from overloading on energy and experiencing the unhealthy conditions associated with unstable blood sugar levels. Fiber slows the release of energy to the body and thus helps avoid the conditions that lead to obesity and diabetes.

"Although genetics may make a person susceptible to diabetes, a diet high in refined, processed foods and low in fiber and complex carbohydrates is believed to be behind most cases of the disease." [17]

Fiber continues to perform duties within the human body. All that wrapping material that filled up the stomach and kept us from overindulging goes on to work more magic. The digestive process extracts antioxidants intermixed in the fiber of fruit and vegetables. The undigested part of fiber continues through the intestines and colon. Like tiny scrub brushes, fiber cleans the gut of toxins and undigested food.

"A high fiber diet also reduces the risk of colon cancer, perhaps by speeding the rate at which stool passes through the intestine and by keeping the digestive tract clean." [18]

Principle Four: Replace Bad Fats with Good Fats

Hunter/gatherers had a substantial amount of fat in their diet. They had to eat like the wild creatures around them. These wild creatures ate wild plants, or ate wild creatures that ate wild plants, or ate wild creatures that ate other wild creatures. As we can see, all forms of life back then contained the ingredients found in the green, leafy plants of the day. Believe it or not, green, leafy, wild plants have small amounts of fat in them. The fats in these plants are called omega-3 fatty acids.

"Omega-3 fatty acids are concentrated in the green leaves of plants (and a few seeds and nuts such as flaxseed, rapeseed, and walnuts)..." [19]

Omega-3 fatty acids are in many plants, but many grains and seeds contain larger amounts of a fatty acid called omega-6.

"... omega-6 fatty acids are mostly concentrated in the seeds and grains, newcomers to our diet." [20]

The ratio of omega-6 to omega-3 EFAs (Essential Fatty Acids) that we have in our diet is particularly significant.

"A critical finding is that your body functions best when your diet contains a balanced ratio of EFAs, yet the typical Western diet contains approximately fourteen to twenty times more omega-6 fatty acids than omega-3." [21]

Grains and corn, the primary feed for most of the livestock that modern man eats, contain high ratios that favor omega-6. Many of today's cooking oils reflect this same imbalance. Some oils have ratios as high as 20:1. For every twenty parts omega-6, there is only one part omega-3. This imbalance of omega fatty acids in the western diet is "linked" to obesity and many diseases that plague modern man.

"Clearly, if you want to fight disease and enjoy optimal health, you need to be eating the ratio of EFAs that sends cancer-fighting, heart-healthy messages to your genes. The ratio that sends those messages studies have shown is a ratio of omega-6 to omega-3 fatty acids that are less than 4 to 1. Not by coincidence, this is similar to the ratio found in our evolutionary diet." [22]

Increasing the ratio of omega-3 in a diet has the added benefit of helping a person lose weight.

"Omega-3 fatty acids also have the ability to enhance thermogenesis, the all-important process by which the body burns fat to produce energy and heat. Thus, the higher percentage of omega-3s you consume, the more you elevate your fat-burning power." [23]

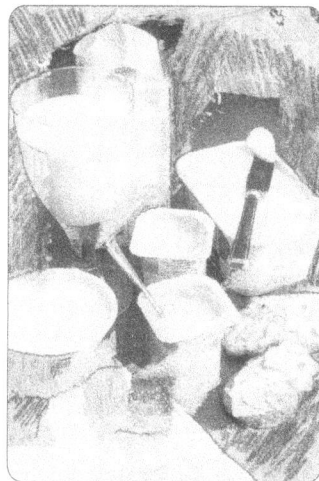

High heat and the refining process produce man-altered products, such as trans fats and hydrogenated oils. These culprits raise bad cholesterol in the body.

Alongside these man-altered fats, are the fats high in saturates. Interestingly, we tend to consume these bad fats and shy away from monounsaturated fats (good fats), found in avocados, nuts, and olive oil.

"Some fatty acids, however, are good for your health. Monounsaturated fatty acids, the type found in olive oil and canola oil, help protect your cardiovascular system. They also reduce the risk of certain metabolic disorders such as insulin resistance and diabetes, and are linked with a lower rate of cancer." [24]

The solution to the "bad fat" dilemma is very easy. We need to replace the bad fats with good fats. We need to replace some of omega-6 intake with omega-3. We need to replace trans fats, hydrogenated oils, and most of saturated fat intake with monounsaturated fats. We need to supplement with food products, which contain omega-6, omega-3 EFAs that reflect the ideal ratio of 3:1.

The Food Cornerstone

Much of the obesity epidemic that plagues America and the developed nations of the world can be traced back to a lack of understanding, or disregard of these principles of nutrition we have discussed.

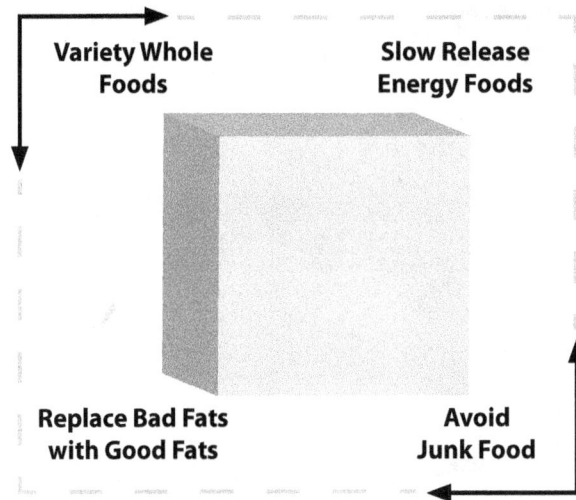

Let us provide a visual image **(Figure 21)**, to help us remember these four principles.

In opposite corners, we start with two principles one is positive (Eat a Variety of Whole Foods), and one is a negative (Avoid Junk food).

As we analyze these two principles, it is clear that they are each connected to the remaining two principles, the replacing principles.

Figure 21: The Food Cornerstone - As we live the principles of eating a variety of food and avoiding junk food, we will gravitate towards foods that are more natural and less processed.

As we live the principle of eating a variety of whole foods, we will gravitate towards foods that are less processed and more natural. Likewise, as we avoid junk food, we gravitate towards foods that are more natural and less processed.

The resulting visual image created by these four principles is a square or rectangle. We will call this geometric shape "The Food Cornerstone." A cornerstone, as many know, is an important structural element to the foundation of a block or stone building. Likewise, by following the four principles discussed, a person will create a strong nutrition cornerstone that will not only help them manage their weight, but also act as a foundation for better health and vitality.

Evolution of the Food Pyramid—Earliest Gatherers

It might surprise some to know that the "Food Pyramid" has not always looked like it presently appears. In fact, originally the Food Pyramid was not a pyramid at all. Rather it looked more like the configuration in the next visual **(Figure 22)**.

This figure shows two triangles within a rectangle. The medium shaded triangle represents gathered food items while the top light shaded triangle reflects hunted meat items.

Section A, located at the very base of the rectangle, represents the diets of the earliest human ancestors. If the theory of evolution is correct, then these creatures were monkeys or monkey like creatures. Like present day monkeys we can assume that their diets consisted of green leafy plants, fruits and vegetables.

Food Profile: Earliest Gatherers

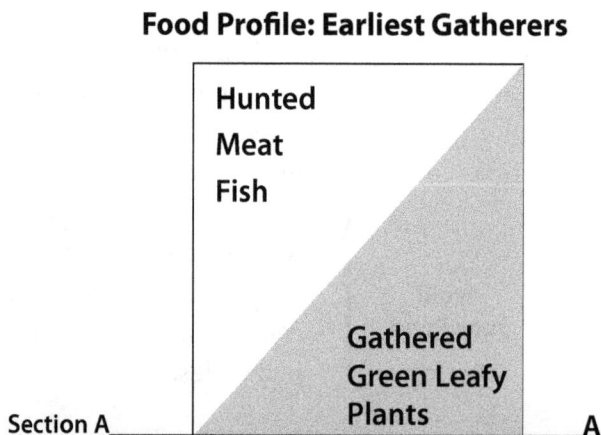

Figure 22: Food Profile: Earliest Gatherers - The earliest gatherer's diet is reflected by Section A. As the section line suggest, their diet consisted of gathered items such as green leafy plants, vegetables, fruits and nuts.

You are what you eat:

Just about everyone has heard this old saying. There is much wisdom in this thought. Our physical body is very forgiving and has the ability to regenerate. The principles of the Nutrition Cornerstone, when combined with the other elements of the "Bases Loaded Program" have the power to change our physical and emotional "being," towards health and vitality.

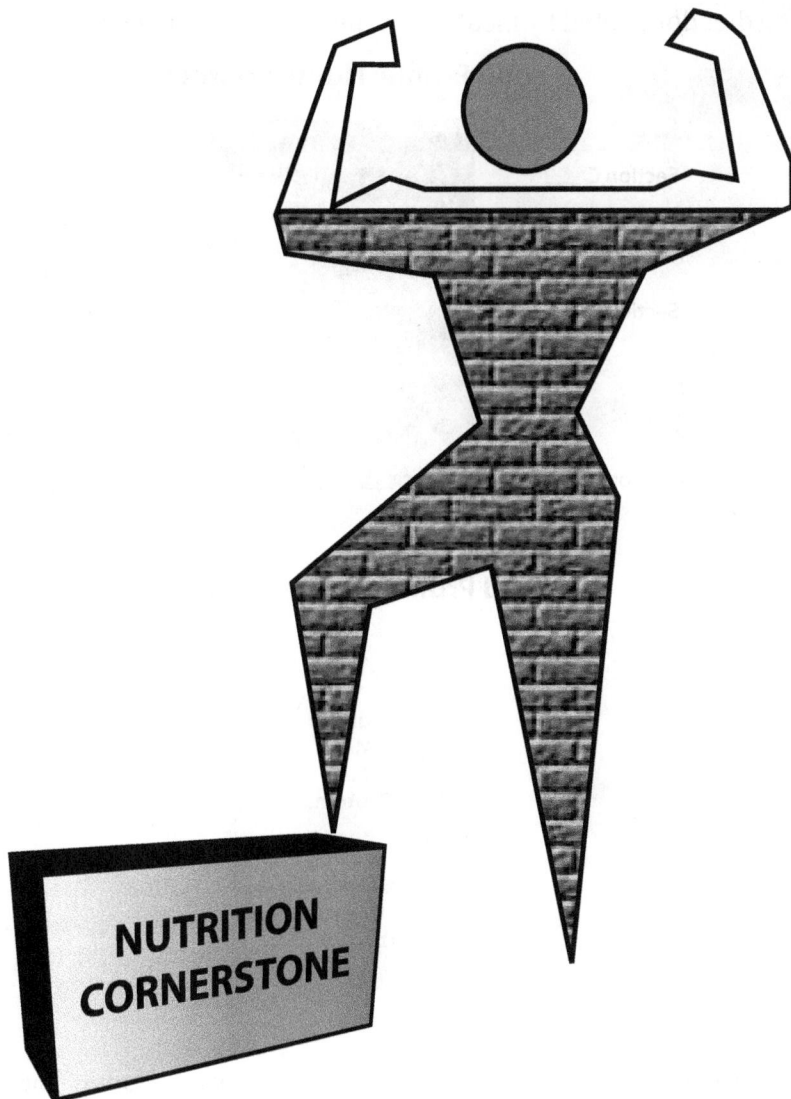

Evolution of the Food Pyramid — Hunter/Gatherers, Egyptians

At some point in the evolutionary development of these creatures, they figured out how to create tools to hunt animals and eat meat. To show this change in diet **(Figure 23)**, we have darkened the triangle labeled "Hunted Meat."

The next section, section B **(Figure 23)**, is moveable. It adjusts up and down the rectangle. Following the dashed line of section B from left to the right, notice that it passes through slightly more medium shade than dark shade. When meat was plentiful, section B would move upwards, reflecting more dark shade, or meat in the diet. Section C, therefore, reflects a diet dominated by meat. If, on the other hand, meat were scarce, section B would

Food Profile: Hunter/Gatherers

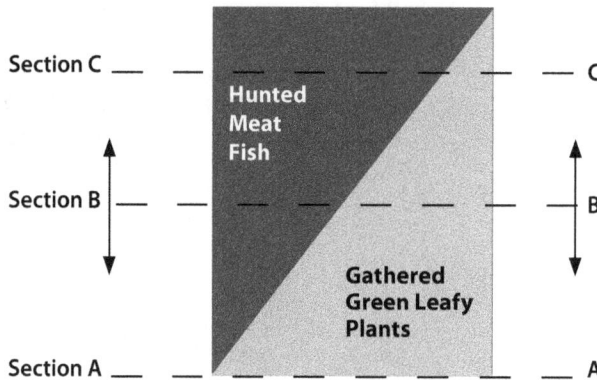

Food Profile: Ancient Egyptians

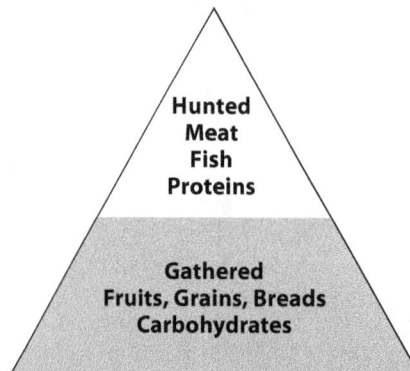

Figure 23: Food Profiles of the Ancient Hunter/Gatherers and the Ancient Egyptians - The Ancient Egyptians transformed the flexible food profile of the hunter/gatherers into a profile where carbohydrates were the main staple of food.

move downward, reflecting more medium shade, or "gathered" food items. For millions of years, the hunter/gatherers' food profile moved within the context of this system (two triangles within a rectangle).

This all changed with the advent of civilization, when people became farmers. The ancient Egyptian culture reflects this change. Those Egyptians not only built tangible pyramids, but unknowingly oriented their eating patterns to pyramids, as well.

Civilization produced a food system that insured the human species' survival. The negative side of that was the fact that it forced a hierarchy to occur within a once flexible food system. Human beings began to obtained most of their fuel from a small variety of carbohydrates, which in turn, compromised their health.

"According to today's "high carbs is best" myth, the Egyptians should have been healthier and more fit. However, that's not the way it worked out. They actually became an obese society with widespread heart disease, stunted growth, and malnutrition." [25]

Today`s Western Diet

"Today's Western diet is the product of industrialization based on inventions ranging from Jethro Tull's seed drill (...to the high speed steel roller mills for milling cereals in the nineteenth century) and advances in processing food to give it a longer shelf life." [26]

"Today's staple carbohydrate foods, including ordinary bread, are quickly digested and absorbed. The resulting effect on blood sugar levels has created a problem for many of us ...much of our diet today is an undesirable but delicious combination of both fat and quickly digested carbohydrate." [27]

America's modernization began in the 1800's and accelerated after the civil war. Like the Egyptians, modern diets eventually evolved into a "pyramid" pattern.

The "Food Pyramid" came out in visual form during the 1990's. It is important to note that the Food Pyramid is an "ideal" representation of the way modern man should eat. We have not drawn up this "ideal" pyramid, but most probably remember it from school. It looks similar to the Egyptian pyramid but divides food into four levels.

The "ideal" pyramid breaks the Egyptian foundation level into two levels. Grains, cereals, bread, and pasta compose the bottom level of the pyramid. The next level up is the fruit and vegetable level. The "ideal" pyramid also breaks the top level of the Egyptian pyramid into two levels. Meats and dairy comprise the third level with fats, oils, and simple sugars being the top level.

Unfortunately, the "reality" of western man's eating patterns and diet, are very different from the experts' perception of the ideal.

The next visual **(Figure 24)** represents Joe's food profile before the Bases Loaded Program. Unfortunately, it is probably a more realistic representation of the actual "modern day" western diet as practiced by children. If I had to choose between the "ideal" and the "more realistic," I would choose the first. Still, I believe there is a better way than all of the pyramids we have discussed.

The Bases Loaded Food Profile:

The "myriad of food pyramids" that shaped civilization has obscured the ideal relationship that we once had with food. The BL-Food Profile **(Figure 25)**, takes us back to the basic root relationship that human beings had with food. Like the ancient hunter/gatherer profile, the new model juxtaposes two triangles within a rectangle. We can compare this relationship to a marriage where the bride and groom represent "Proteins" and "Unrefined Carbohydrates" respectively (grooms are usually more unrefined). A happy marriage recognises the equal worth of both male and female. Both have qualities and characteristics that complement and build the other, and thus each separate half has equal validity. Whenever we try to put one entity over another by saying that one is more important or of more worth than the other, we no longer have a marriage, but rather a hierarchy. Where do we human beings fit into this analogy? We are the "children" of the marriage. There are times and seasons of life where the children need the touch of the mother. There are other times when children need the touch of the father. So it is with the food triangles. There are times when we will need to emphasize the protein triangle, and other times when we will need to emphasize the unrefined carbohydrates triangle. Neither triangle, however, should be ignored. For they both provide nourishment and are of equal worth.

A Diet that Mimics the Hunter/Gatherer Diet

The Bases Loaded Program advocates balance and variety rather than hierarchy. The visual representation of the BL-Program, looks much like the visual representation of the hunter/gatherer profile. It is a "slow release" energy model like the original model, but slightly modified.

Unlike ancient ancestors, people in developed nations actively control their diet. The profile has a "Zone of Balance" represented by the dashed lines. A person who orients their food profile within this zone will find a balance between the two triangles. A person

Food Profile: Joe - Before Bases Loaded Program

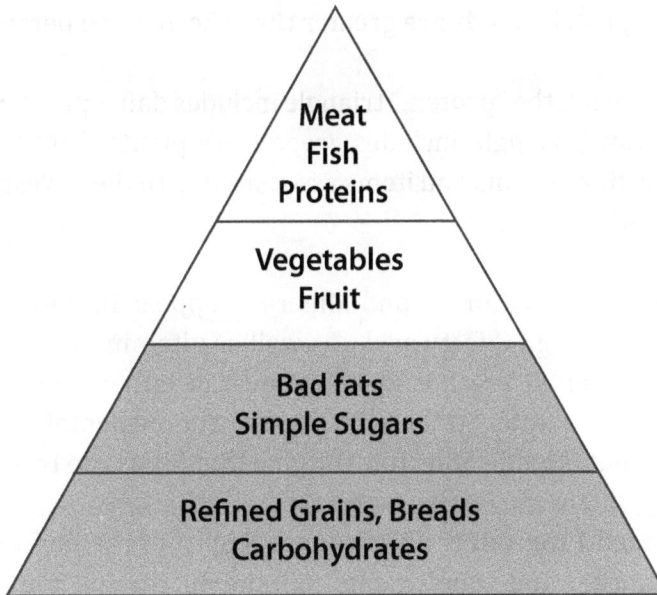

Meat
Fish
Proteins

Vegetables
Fruit

Bad fats
Simple Sugars

Refined Grains, Breads
Carbohydrates

Figure 24: Food Profile: Joe - Before Bases Loaded Program - Joe's food profile before the BL-Program is indicative of today's western diet, where the foundation foods are unhealthy.

The Bases Loaded Food Profile

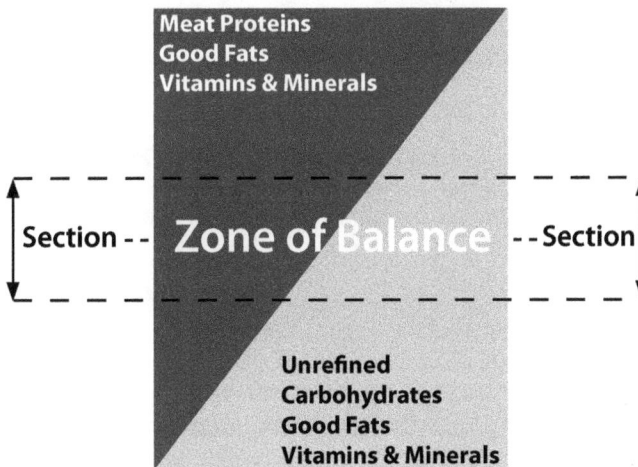

Meat Proteins
Good Fats
Vitamins & Minerals

Section -- Zone of Balance -- Section

Unrefined
Carbohydrates
Good Fats
Vitamins & Minerals

Figure 25: The Bases Loaded Food Profile - The BL-Plan advocates a food profile that mimics the ancient hunter/gatherer profile, where one is nourished by a healthy balance of proteins, carbohydrates, good fats, vitamins and minerals.

has the flexibility to move up or down within this zone, according to their needs. Athletes and physically active people who use their muscles in their work would be situated at the top of the zone. Their protein needs are greater than the average person.

In addition to fish and meat, the "protein" triangle includes dairy, poultry, meat substitutes while the "carbohydrate" triangle includes green leafy plants, fruits and vegetables, as well as the whole unrefined grains and items associated with the lowest level of the "ideal" pyramid discussed earlier.

Notice the label "Good Fats, Vitamins and Minerals" appear in both triangles. This has to do with the fact that omega-3 fatty acids, as well as vitamins and minerals, (including antioxidants, trace elements) are not in abundance in either modern day triangle as they were in the original hunter/gatherer triangles. Supplementation then becomes an important part of the nutrition profile. It is the glue that binds the triangles together.

While the Bases Loaded Program is not an exact replica of the hunter/gatherer profile, through wise food choices and supplementation, the nutritional content of the modern day diet can mimic that of the hunter/gatherer ancestors.

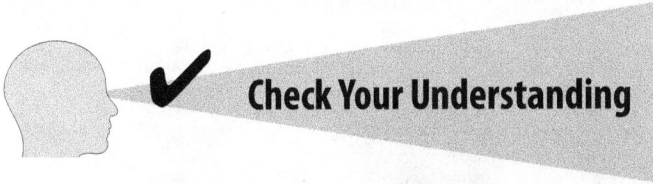

Check Your Understanding

1. **What are the four principles that comprise the Food Cornerstone?**

   Answer: *The four principles comprising the Food Cornerstone are; Eat a Variety of Food, Avoid Junk Food, Replace Quick Release Energy Foods with Slow Release Energy Foods, and Replace Bad Fats with Good Fats.*

2. **Is it true that diets advocating the eating of one type of healthy food help us to lose weight?**

   Answer: *In the short-term, restrictive diets will cause the body to lose weight, but these types of diets lead to weight gain in the long-term.*

3. **From Mr. Metabolism's perspective, why do human beings love the taste of sugar and fat?**

   Answer: *The love for fat and sugar is instinctual because these types of food are energy commodities.*

4. **What is the natural packing material contained in unrefined energy food?**

   Answer: *Fiber is nature's packing material.*

5. **What is the ideal ratio of omega-6 to omega-3?**

   Answer: *The ideal ratio is 3:1.*

6. **When it comes to proteins and carbohydrates, is the BL-Food Profile based upon the principle of hierarchy or balance?**

   Answer: *The BL-Food Profile advocates a healthy balance of protein and carbohydrates.*

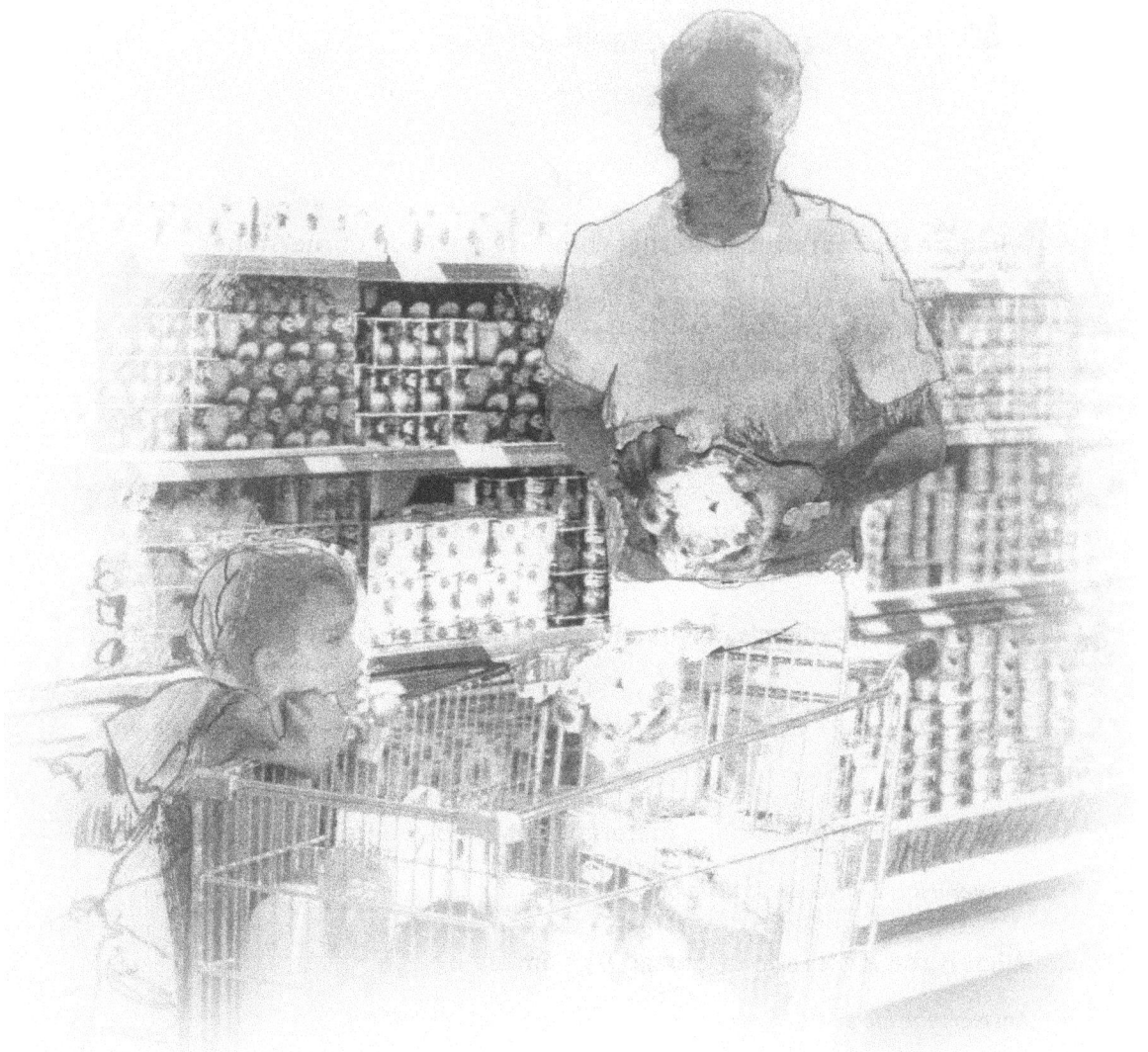

Unlike the hunter/gatherers, we face predators of beautifully wrapped packages of processed food that can compromise our family's health.

Going Shopping

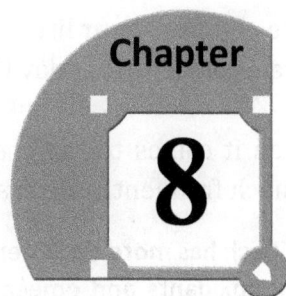

Fortunately, for us, the rule that applied to the hunter/gatherer ancestors applies to modern man: "The hunter must be smarter than his prey." Ancestor hunters had to be smarter than the deer or antelope. Modern man needs to be at least as smart as a free-range chicken or a can of tuna fish. We have the advantage!

Let us take a trip to the grocery store and incorporate the principles of the "Food Cornerstone" into the buying. We will first want to visit the vegetable section of the store. As we all know, the vegetable section is the place where they keep the green leafy stuff, the food hunter/gatherers ate.

Fruits and Vegetables

At the fruit and vegetable section, pause a moment and look at the variety of shapes and colors. Ever noticed that some of the happiest workers in the grocery store work in the produce section? I think it is because of color and beauty that surrounds them.

It goes without saying that we will make friends with these produce workers since we will see them more often than many family relatives. Always visit this section first. Feel free to visit this section of the store every few days. Over the years, you should wear a path in the floor, from the front entrance of the store to the produce section.

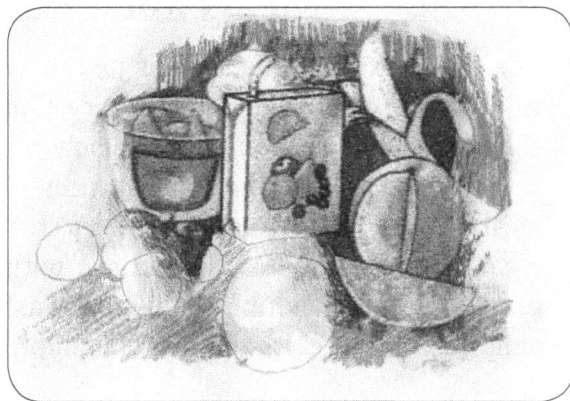

Most snack items will come from the produce section of the store. Grapes, oranges, melons, cut-up apples, strawberries, kiwi, bananas, fresh cut-up pineapple, all make great snacks. Children love to eat cherry tomatoes, baby carrots, cut-up celery, snap peas, broccoli, and red peppers. Soon the happiness of the produce section will be reflected in the faces of your little children. Your little ones will think they have the greatest mom or dad in the world because every other day they get a box full of colorful food that tastes good.

When it comes to the green leafy stuff, I always think of Joe's Uncle Popeye who eats spinach frequently. He is a strong man.

"Spinach has more documented health benefits than almost any other food. Beyond its supplies of antioxidants and omega-3s, it is an important source of coenzyme Q10, which is vital to cellular energy production and fat burning." [28]

The thing I like about spinach is the price. Even though, it is one of the healthiest foods, it is also one of the least expensive! Feel free to get spinach and other types of dark green leafy vegetables. Make tasty salads using these dark leafy greens as your base ingredients.

Take a moment before leaving the produce section to take a look at your fellow shoppers. Ever noticed that some of the happiest shoppers in the grocery store congregate in the produce section? Why is this? These people are happy because they are fulfilling their most basic instinctual urge to "gather" the same types of food the hunter/gatherers gathered.

Proteins—Meats and Poultry

The next section of the store is just as valuable to us as the produce section. Notice that the shoppers in this section are extremely serious shoppers. They, like the hunter ancestors of old, take their job very seriously. They stalk the meat, poultry, and seafood sections with cell phone in hand consulting their wife or husband at home as to the catch they are contemplating.

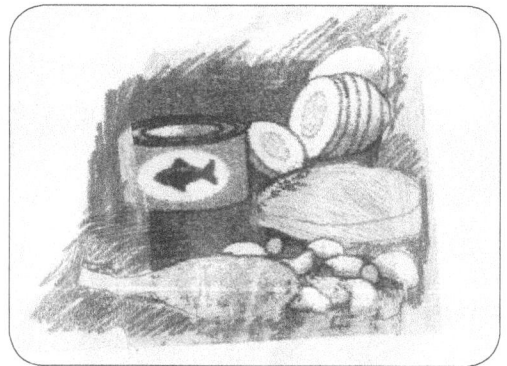

I take a relaxed approach to find meat for meals. Since meat, like produce, is a plentiful thing, I do not have to worry about my family starving as I am sure the hunter/gatherers worried. I do my meat shopping according to the bargains. Unlike my ancestors of old, I have a deep freezer at home where I can store meat bargains for days to come.

When it comes to meat, my family likes variety. I divide my meats into six categories. They are red meat, white meat, brown meat, seafood, B&B, and meat substitutes.

Red meat includes lean beef, lean hamburger, steak-trimmed of fat, and yes, buffalo meat on occasion. White meat includes chicken, turkey, and turkey bacon. Brown meat includes ham and thick pork steaks trimmed of fat. Seafood includes all types of "wild caught" fish. Tuna fish, sardines, and salmon are the most common fish that my family eats. Occasionally we eat shrimp. Seafood is particularly important for the omega-3 oil it contains. As discussed earlier, omega-3 oil is important for the body, but it also plays an essential role in a person's mental health.

B&B refers to brown rice and beans, a popular combination in vegetarian meals. Meat, as most people know is a good source of protein. What many people do not know is that when eaten together, brown rice and beans combine to make a complete protein, equal to the complete protein found in meat.

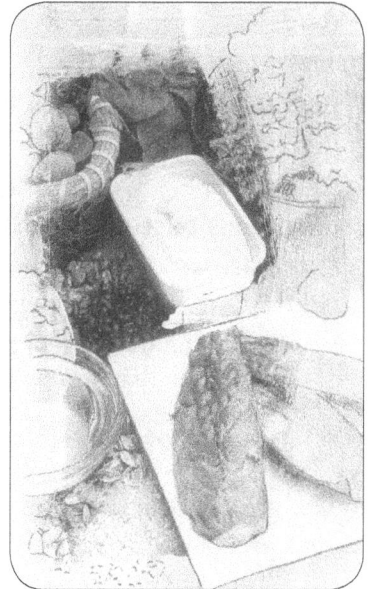

There are other sources of complete proteins that we will categorize as meat substitutes. These include tofu, omega eggs, low fat yogurt, low fat cheese, cottage cheese and nuts.

These visits to produce and meat sections have in large part fulfilled the #1 nutrition principle. Incorporating more fruits and vegetables into meals, as well as seafood and lean meats will in most cases bring variety and balance to the average American diet. Perhaps we will fool Mr. Metabolism into believing that we really are hunter/gatherers!

Sadly, we will leave these sections of the grocery store where we shop using instincts. We must now shop in some sections where we have to use eyes, brains and willpower. Willpower? How do we use willpower? See those doughnuts over there, smell the freshly baked French bread? Pass them by. Do not be enticed by them. Put your blinders on. Remember your nutrition principles and search for better options.

Good Fats

Before we forget, there is an essential supplement we must buy. A significant ingredient is missing from store bought meat.

Today's meat is severely deficient in omega-3 fatty acids. Let us restore the healthy balance of 3:1, omega-6 to omega-3. Swing by the supplement section of the store and buy some flax oil and fish oil capsules.

Replace regular eggs with eggs that advertise a higher content of omega-3. Replace butter with a buttery spread, but here is where one must use their eyes and brain. Look carefully at the contents of the spread. Avoid margarines that have hydrogenated oils or trans-fats. There are some buttery spreads that advertise a high content of omega-3 fatty acids. These are the ones to buy.

Other items to look for that contain high amounts of omega-3 fatty acids include certain types of mayonnaise, pumpkin seeds, walnuts, walnut oil, and "cold pressed" canola oil. If your grocery store does not have some of these items, most health food stores do.

In addition to getting food items containing omega-3 fatty acids, we will need to buy food rich in monounsaturated fats. Buy "extra virgin" olive oil. Be liberal with it in your low temperature cooking, baking, and salads. Other sources of monounsaturated fats include avocado, and 100% natural peanut butter. Buy some mixed nuts and add to these, walnuts, pumpkin seeds, almonds, carob pieces, dates or raisins to make a nutritious snack mix.

Okay shoppers, we have saved the trickiest part of shopping for last. Before beginning this dangerous part of the mission, look down at your shopping cart. Your hunter/gatherer ancestors would be proud of your efforts. Your cart is full of meat, fruit, vegetables and good fats. True, your ancestors would not recognize the packaging in some cases, but they sure would enjoy the feast these food items provide.

Carbohydrates

The next part of the shopping excursion is tricky because once again, one must use their eyes and brains to sift out the imposters. It is dangerous because there are predators out there. Unlike the hunter/gatherers, we face predators of beautifully wrapped packages of processed food that can compromise our family's health.

The next part of the mission is to shop for carbohydrates or "energy food." True, digestion breaks down all food to provide energy to the body. Some foods, though, such as "refined carbohydrates," raise the blood sugar level quickly, and overwhelm the body with energy. Ironically, such foods rob the body of energy.

When these foods become part of the family diet, over time, they can lead to obesity and a myriad of health problems.

The shopping cart already has many good unrefined carbohydrates in it. These include fruits and vegetables. They are natures "energy foods." They will bring energy and other vital nutrients to the body quicker than meat or "good fats." On the other hand, their delivery of energy will be much slower than refined carbohydrates.

The remaining task once again is to use the nutrition principles from the "Food Cornerstone" as a guide. Let us avoid junk food, sift through the counterfeits, and choose "slow energy release food" over "quick energy release food."

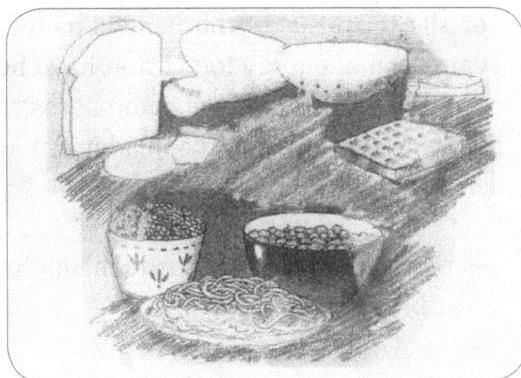

Glycemic Index

There is another tool that will be helpful in the next part of the shopping excursion. Most shoppers have probably heard of the Glycemic Index. It is an index used to help people distinguish between slow, moderate, and quick energy release foods. The slowest energy release food would be given the number 1. The quickest energy release food would be given the number 100.

We do not need to evaluate the foods that we have gathered thus far using the Glycemic Index. Just about all fruits and vegetables, meats and fats have a low index. There are exceptions to the rule. The important thing to keep in mind, is that for people who do not have certain medical conditions, the health benefits associated with these exceptions far outweigh their high GI rating.

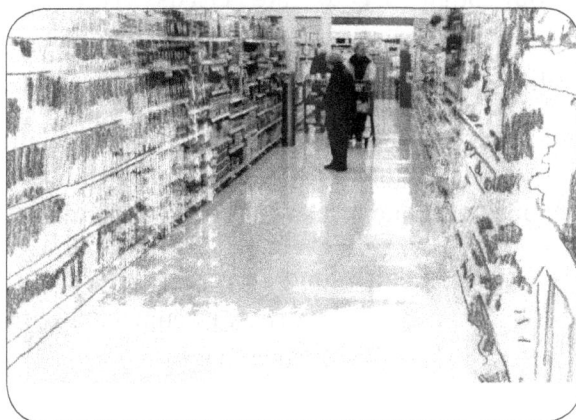

The Glycemic Index is an invaluable tool for those who are diabetic or borderline diabetic. Such an index empowers patients and their physicians to make wise choices concerning the patient's diet. Herein we find another important reason for checking with your doctors before implementing the Bases Loaded Program. This program allows for food that might be "off limits" for your situation. Perhaps your family doctor will offer some modifications to the program in regards to food.

For the purposes of the Bases Loaded Plan, the Glycemic Index is a helpful tool in the evaluation of energy foods that have been "processed" to certain degrees by the hand of man. We will sometimes come across a food item that advertises itself as having a low glycemic index. We will consider any food item, indexed 50 or less, to be a slow energy release food item.

Get ready for a whirlwind ride through the remaining aisles of the supermarket. First stop is the bread aisle.

Bread Aisle

Stay away from white bread. White bread means white flour. White flour means highly refined. Look for bread marked 100% stone ground wheat.

When it comes to wheat bread, I like to use the balancing arm test. Pick up two different brands of equal size wheat bread and compare weight. Usually the heavier bread is less refined and, therefore, the better pick. It might cost more, but the taste and health benefits are worth it.

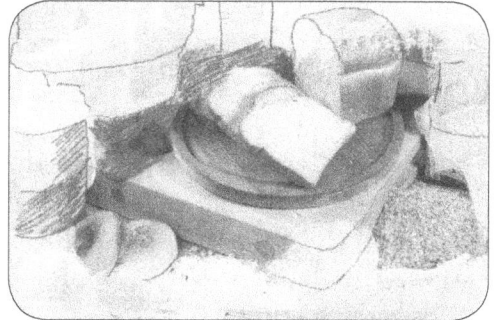

Sourdough breads are also good. Cracked wheat sourdough bread is one of Joe's favorites. Sourdough bread, like citrus fruit or most spicy food, slows the release of sugars from the stomach.

"Sourdough breads, in which lactic acid and propionic acid are produced by the natural fermentation of starch and sugars by the yeast starter culture, also produce reduced levels of blood sugar and insulin compared with normal bread." [29]

Go to the health food store and check out their breads. There are also specialty bread stores that have healthy alternatives to the fluffy variety of breads that dominate the bread aisle of the supermarket.

Spreads for the Bread

Buy 100% peanut butter or almond butter with no added sugar or hydrogenated oil. Buy jelly, which contains, 100% fruit with no added sugar or sweeteners. These spreads allow one to make healthy sandwiches and snacks.

Flour and Basic Cooking Materials

Whole oats are better than quick oats. Buy flour, that is 100% stone ground whole wheat for your pancakes or waffles. Buckwheat is a nutritious food item that is excellent for pancakes or waffles. Used in combination with 100% stone ground wheat, buckwheat will produce a finer textured result for baked items. Wheat germ, cracked wheat, oat bran and wheat bran are also important ingredients for the fiber they contain, and can be used in a variety of recipes.

Simple Sugars

Before we pick anything up from this aisle, it must be said that the Bases Loaded Program will reduce your simple sugar intake drastically. The problem with simple sugar is that it takes away the appetite for other types of food, thus depriving the body of essential food combinations. We want to stay away from all the drinks and snacks loaded with sugar and corn syrup. The simple sugars we suggest should be used sparingly. For the most part, they should be used in healthy desserts that the family makes occasionally.

Having said that, there is an important item to pick up at the health food store. It is a natural sweetener made from the Agave plant. It comes in liquid syrup form. Some brands advertise this product as having a particularly low glycemic index. We use it to sweeten plain yogurt, or make cinnamon toast. There are different brand names with slightly different tastes. Find it near the honey section.

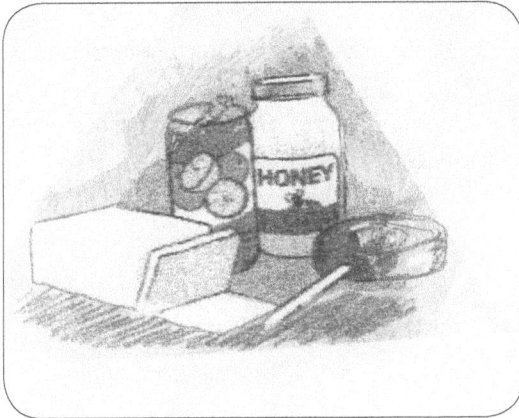

Replace white sugar and corn syrup with honey, molasses, date sugar, and 100% maple sugar or maple syrup. It should be noted that small infants should not have honey as it may contain spores that could be harmful to their health. White sugar and corn syrup are highly refined carbohydrates. Their replacements are less refined than white sugar and corn syrup.

Honey and molasses, dates, raisins, and 100% maple syrup have another advantage. Refined sugars acidify the body, sometimes leading to a condition known as acidosis.

"Acidosis is a condition in which body chemistry becomes imbalanced and overly acidic...eat alkaline-forming foods (such as)...Avocados, Corn, Fresh Coconut, Most Fresh Fruit, Most Grains, Honey, Maple Syrup, Molasses, Raisins, Soy Products." [30]

It seems that many who are overweight or obese develop acidosis.

"Acidosis occurs when the body loses its alkaline reserve. Some causes of acidosis include... obesity," [31]

This condition is particularly hard on the joints as any person with arthritis can testify. Honey, molasses, dates, raisins, and 100% maple syrup, on the other hand, help to reduce acidity and balance pH.

Juice

Surprisingly, another food item that helps reduce acidity and pH are the citrus fruits, such as oranges, grapefruits and tangerines.

"Although it might seem that citrus fruits would have an acidifying effect on the body, the citric acid they contain actually has an alkalinizing effect in the system." [32]

Those that like orange juice or grapefruit juice are in luck. These juices have the added benefit of slowing the absorption from the stomach.

"The low glycemic index of grapefruit may be due to their high acid content which slows absorption from the stomach." [33]

"Well known as a good source of vitamin C, most of the sugar content of oranges is sucrose. This and their high acid content, probably accounts for their low G. I." [34]

Dairy

A few more items will round out the breakfast and snack foods. Buy low fat milk. Skim milk is best, but buy the low fat milk your family enjoys the most. Low fat cream cheese, cottage cheese, string cheese, plain low fat yogurt and low fat sour cream are also items to buy.

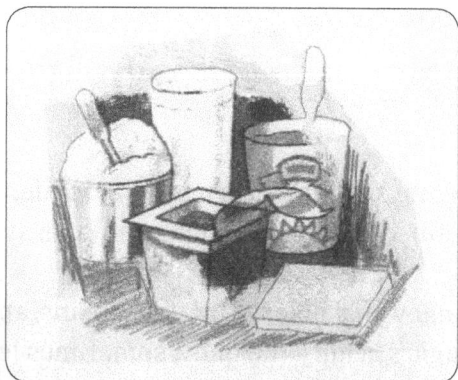

Tasty snacks can be made using cream cheese or string cheese with crackers and pickles. Look carefully at labels. Be sure your crackers are 100% whole grain and high in fiber. Use the "loud sound" test when choosing crackers. The louder the sound that a cracker makes when chewed, the better! Look at the label and notice that the loudest crackers usually contain the most fiber.

Cereals

When choosing cereal, remember, less refined is better. High fiber cereals, oatmeal (the kind that cooks up in five minutes as opposed to one minute), are the types of cereals to get. Add some Agave syrup and or fresh fruit to sweeten them.

Unfortunately, most cereal products fall in the category of highly refined carbohydrates, or junk food. The best cereals are homemade cereals. Find a granola recipe that your family loves. As with all recipes, use the "replacement principles" of the Food Cornerstone to transform the granola recipe into a healthier recipe.

Snack Items

Make fruit puree by blending frozen berries with a small jar of 100% fruit jelly, Agave syrup, and a little water. This puree mixture makes a fabulous snack or dessert when put over fruit, yogurt or cottage cheese. Low fat sour cream and salsa are invaluable materials for dips and toppings for meals. Mix these two items with black beans, pinto beans, or mashed up avocados for a nutritious dip. Plain corn chips that are 100% corn, light on the oil are the type of chips your family will need to accompany a nutritious dip.

Odds and Ends for Meals

Basic meal items include lean ham and turkey lunch meat, low fat cheese, onions, chicken and beef broth. Beans, lentils, and peas are super fiber foods to use in your meals. These basic items, in combination with breakfast and snack items already mentioned will allow for a variety of soup and sandwich meals.

Dinner Carbohydrates

Complex carbohydrates differ from simple sugars in that their sugar chains are longer or more "complex" than simple sugars. These are the types of carbohydrates that we should be getting daily. In their whole state, they provide a slow sustained release of energy to the body. Since we should be incorporating these carbohydrates into meals, I call them "dinner carbohydrates." Feel free to eat them at any meal. I divide dinner carbohydrates into five categories. They are potatoes, pasta, rice, corn or yams, and the "catchall category."

The "catchall category" includes ethnic specialties like Quinoa and couscous. It also includes vegetables, whole grains, peas, squash, lentils, and beans. Within each of these categories, there are many types. Here again is where the Glycemic Index can help us. For example, there are many types of rice, but my family uses parboiled or brown rice, because the glycemic indexes of these two, are lower compared to other types of rice commonly found in the grocery store.

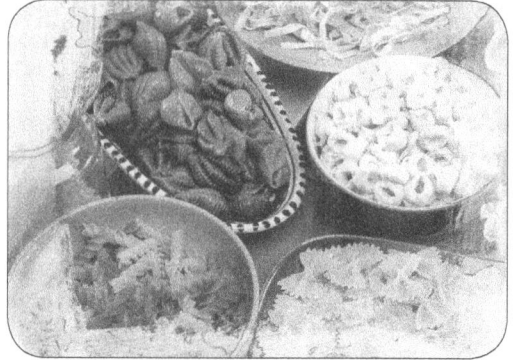

These carbohydrates are essential sources of energy and when eaten with proteins and vegetables, provide invaluable food combinations for your family. When eaten with their skins, or eaten in their whole state, they become good sources of fiber, and other nutrients. Try eating a baked potato with its skin. Eat it with some low fat sour cream and onions or chives and be surprised how good it tastes.

On the way Home

That truly was a whirlwind tour! I probably missed a few things, but just remember the nutrition principles contained in the Food Cornerstone, to help make decisions.

Remember to stop by the health food store on the way home. While there, check out the protein bars. I like to include one bar on the snack table for Joe, to be eaten before dinner sometime. Look for protein bars that are high in protein and fiber.

Here is something to keep in mind for the later stages of your child's program. Consider the possibility of a protein supplement. As your child loses weight, the intensity of their nightly workouts will increase. In the latter stages of Joe's program, I got a protein supplement from the health food store. They come in powder form, in a variety of flavors, and can be used to make refreshing shakes.

Check out the aisles in the health food store. Do not be fooled by the label "health" that is attached to a store or a food item. There are predators mixed in with the good no matter where one shops. Practice wise hunter/gatherer principles whenever shopping and your family will be happy eaters!

Daydream Dinner

Simmer leftover vegetables from the snack bar, in chicken or beef broth. To add extra flavor to the broth and vegetables, add a can of low fat soup.

Cook a scrambled egg with cut up pieces of ham or turkey lunchmeat. Include some cheese, leafy vegetables, tomato, grated Parmesan cheese and avocado for a nutritious sandwich. Flavor your meat and vegetable sandwiches with a mixture of mayonnaise, mustard, and a little amount of vinegar for a tangy taste.

Need More Variety?

Notice that I broke meats into six categories and carbohydrates into five categories. I did this for a reason. I have found that a significant challenge facing the person preparing meals, is to feed the family a variety of food.

Busy schedule and financial constraints usually restrict creative thinking when it comes to dinners. We figure out a few meals that the family will eat, and we tend to make these same meals weekly without any variety. Here is a proven method to help bring variety to your meals. Make yourself a chart that has two lists. Number the meat categories, one through six. Label the carbohydrate categories a through e. We will use these categories to plan meals for the coming weeks. These meals will be for the workdays, Monday through Friday. We will designate Saturday as leftover day, and Sunday as a "cook whatever you want" day. Start with the first category for each of these food types. So your first Monday night will be (1a), red meat and potatoes. Night two will be (2b), white meat and pasta. Continue this chart by not varying the order of your respective categories. Because your meat category has one more category than your carbohydrate category, it will take 31 matches to get back to (1a), red meat and potatoes pairing up again.

Excluding Saturday and Sunday, this translates into six working weeks of dinner variety for your meats and carbohydrates. Using this method, the only thing we have to think about during the day is what vegetables we need to include with the meal!

Do your Children Need More Meat and Vegetables?

All of my children, including Joe, are picky eaters. Here are some ideas on how to incorporate meats and vegetables into your meals. What is your child's favorite ethnic food? Most ethnic dishes cut meat into small pieces and include them in sauces/soups to be placed over or with the carbohydrate of the meal. Pizza, lasagna, tacos, Indian curry dishes, sweet and sour Chinese dishes all use this basic pattern to create tasty food combinations. Include vegetables into sauces/soups, or melt some low fat cheese over them. Cut up fresh vegetables and serve them with a tangy dip or dressing. Be creative and have fun bringing balance and variety to the meal.

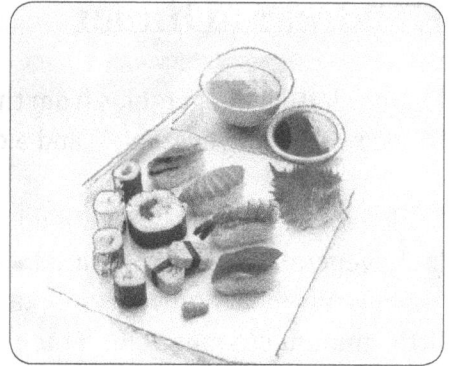

Condiments?

Catsup, sweet pickles and many salad dressings contain sugar. There are two approaches one can use. The expensive approach would be to buy your condiments at the health food store. I take the cheaper route. Regarding food, the BL-Program is 98% healthy and 2% tolerant of junk food. I choose to use condiments that have corn syrup or sugar sparingly, knowing that a little bit can make the difference between children deciding to eat the healthy food that dominates the meal. I have not caught any of my children drinking the salad dressing. On the other hand, Joe overindulges with the catsup on the eggs, but he gets that tradition from me!

Last and Certainly Least... Dessert!

Is it possible to eat dessert within the boundaries of the BL-Program? My short answer is yes. Here is the long answer. By definition, dessert is something sweet that we have at the end of dinner. Fruits and fruit salads make excellent desserts and are desirable foods to end dinner with in the Bases Loaded Program. The challenge with dessert, is the fact that the period immediately after dinner is a critical time where we are trying to cut down on food, and increase physical activity. The last thing we need to do is create the habit of eating sweet desserts at this time. So here is what my family does. I make one sweet dessert per week. On the "rest" day, I make something special like peanut butter cookies, carrot cake, or custard with berries.

I always make sure that this dessert uses ingredients that make it a "slow release energy food." Whole wheat flour, cracked wheat, oatmeal, wheat germ, buckwheat, oat bran and wheat bran replace refined flour. Olive oil and buttery spread enriched with omega-3, replace butter or margarine. Omega-3 enriched eggs replace regular eggs. Honey or Agave syrup replaces refined sugar. In other words, I use the Nutrition Cornerstone "replacement principles" to create healthy desserts. If my family does not eat all of the desert Sunday, then we save it for Monday. During the week, we eat any leftover dessert during the day rather than after dinner. Thus, we only have one dinner a week that is followed by a sweet dessert other than fruit. We try to have the main meal on Sunday at 2:00 or 3:00 p.m. We follow this meal with a family walk and have a snack-sized meal for the last food of the day. Guess what we do after the last food of the day on Sunday? That is right we take another walk.

Activity to Save Money

When it comes to grocery shopping, saving money requires organization. Here a helpful activity that requires an investment of time and energy on the part of those that do the grocery shopping, but the activity is well worth it. Not only will this activity help implement the BL-Food Program in regards to food, but the suggestions offered here will also save the family money in the years to come. Experience has taught me that the price for a particular food item varies from store to store. Along with this idea, grocery stores tend to have certain sections where their prices are lower than their competitors. One store may have the lowest meat prices while another store has the lowest produce prices. To take advantage of the bargains, let us create a list.

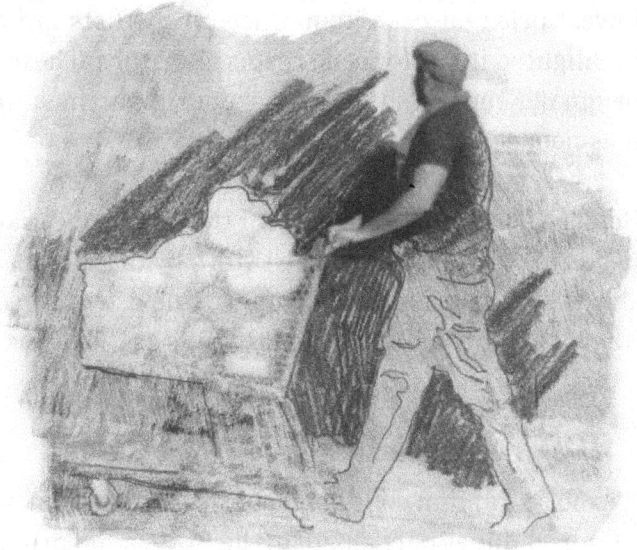

Organize the list under the following headings:

- **Fruits and Vegetables**

- **Meats and poultry**

- **Fats**

- **Carbohydrates**

- **Breads**

- **Spreads for the Bread**

- **Flour and Cooking Materials**

- **Simple Sugars**

- **Juice**

- **Cereals**

- **Dairy**

- **Snack Items**

- **Odds and Ends**

- **Dinner Carbohydrates**

Notice that these headings correspond to the headings of the chapter we just read. Under each heading, list the food items that we discussed in the chapter. Now there should be a few sheets of paper with lists on them. These sheets are originals. Use the originals to generate several copied sets. Label each set with the name of one of the local grocery stores where the family shops. When shopping at a store, take the respective set, and write down the price of each food item listed in the set. This part of the process may require several visits. After completing all the sets, compare them and highlight the lowest price for each item. Once all the lists are highlighted, make a shortlist of all the highlighted items for each respective store. These sheets constitute your shortlist packet original. Keep the shortlist packet original in a safe place and periodically make copies of it as needed.

Before shopping, take a copy of the shortlist packet, and highlight the items your family needs for the week. Visit each store by driving in a big loop that ends back home. Use the shortlist packet as a tool. Compare sale price items, to the respective highlighted shortlist items. Buy the items the family needs at the lowest price, and save.

Food Too Expensive?

It is no secret that childhood obesity is prevalent among lower income families. Can lower income families participate in the BL-Loaded program? Yes they can! In many ways, lower income families in America are no different than higher income families in America. Children rush off to school without eating breakfast. Their days are filled with schoolwork and physical activities, while their evenings are spent resting and refueling.

One of the great messages of this book is that all human beings, no matter what their race, gender, or socioeconomic status, share a common bond. When it comes to the metabolism, we are all made the same way. The principles that govern the metabolism are the same for all human beings. Understanding these principles and learning to work with the metabolism will help one lose weight, just as it helped Joe lose weight! That being said let me offer some practical suggestions for those that do not have a lot of money to spend on food, but desire to implement the BL-Program.

First suggestion: Follow the principles contained in this book regarding the timing of meals and exercise. Ignoring these principles will lead to weight gain, no matter how poor or nutritious the diet.

Second suggestion: Do not try to make all the dietary changes at once. Continue to buy food items that your family enjoys eating, but buy less of the respective items that do not fit within the guidelines of the BL-Program. Take some of the money you save and buy some of the wholesome foods listed in this chapter. I would recommend the following items to get started; 100% whole wheat bread, eggs, turkey bacon, orange juice, olive oil, brown rice and beans.

Third suggestion: Take some of the money that you have saved (from the above suggestion) and buy some important supplements for your family. We will talk more about supplements in the next chapter. In the early stages of the program buy a good multivitamin as well as fish oil capsules. Have your family take these two supplements as outlined in the next chapter.

Fourth suggestion: Continue to expand the variety of wholesome food for your family. Slowly replace the unhealthy food with its respective healthy counterpart.

Elvis Presley and Food

Elvis Presley's favorite snack was peanut butter on white bread. He enjoyed this snack even after he was a famous rock and roll star with millions of dollars. This little piece of trivia teaches an important lesson. The food we eat is connected to something more than money. Food is connected to taste, and taste being a pleasure, is connected to love. Elvis loved his mother. It was his mother that fed him peanut butter sandwiches all those years that their family was poor. It is important to realize this connection between love and food, as we make dietary changes in the family. We are not trying to get rid of the bonds of love that hold the family together, rather expand those bonds of love.

Do not miss the next chapter. Like the food chapters, it contains important information that will help keep your family healthy and strong. Since the food chapters were rather long, stand up and do a few jumping jacks. Do not break a sweat while doing them. Just do enough to keep Mr. Metabolism from going into conservation mode. The small seemingly insignificant body movements that we perform in the course of the day are very significant to the speed Mr. Metabolism chooses to run.

By providing our body the nutrients it needs, both in food and supplements, cravings are eliminated, and our desire for food will follow a much more normal pattern.

Supplements

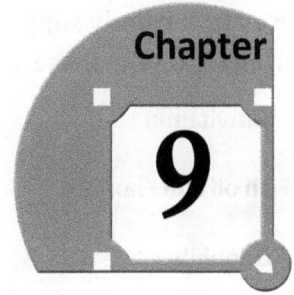

Unfortunately, food is not what it used to be. I lived in Ohio during the first eight years of my life. I can still remember Sunday meals at my grandmother's house. The table was laden with chicken, fresh corn on the cob, hot rolls, green beans, salad, potatoes and lemonade. For dessert, there were fresh picked strawberries or peaches on ice cream. I can still see the image of it all in my mind. Sadly, I cannot remember the taste of the food. For the most part, those particular tastes are now extinct in America.

The source of all food, save seafood, goes back to the soil. We grow vegetables in the soil. Chickens and cows eat plants and grain that come from the soil. Ultimately, it is the combination of sun, water and nutrients in the soil that determine the nutritional profile of the natural food we eat. So what has happened, to the soil in America and other developed nations of the world?

Certainly the sun has not changed, nor has the water. The only other factors then are the nutrients of the soil. America's fertilization practices have leached nutrients from farmland soil. Processing and refinement of food also strips away nutrients. These dramatic changes have manifested themselves in the nutritional content and even the taste of food.

One way to combat this predicament is to grow fruits and vegetables the old fashioned way. Anyone who has kept a garden knows the rewards, both tangible and intangible, of such an endeavor.

Another way to combat this situation is to take a few important supplements daily. While these supplements will not make the present day food taste like the food of 50 years ago, it will help the nutritional profile of the family diet.

Besides helping nutritional status, these recommended supplements play a big part in helping children achieve ideal weight. Remember from previous discussions, "cravings" are a big culprit in the story of weight gain. Proper nutrition eliminates cravings. Without cravings, the desire for food follows a much more normal pattern.

These are the daily supplements Joe took during his program. Since his program, Joe has continued to take these supplements, all save Chromium Picolinate.

- **Multivitamin**

- **Fish oil and Flax oil**

- **Acidophilus**

- **Chromium Picolinate**

- **Glutathione**

The type of multivitamin that your child takes will be different from the one that adults take. Of course, children prefer chewable vitamins. Parents choose a multivitamin suitable for your age and gender. Most health food experts recommend food derived vitamins rather than chemical derived vitamins.

Fish and Flax Oil

As discussed earlier, the food combination of protein/good fats, acted as a nutritional foundation for the hunter/gatherers. To mimic this nutritional foundation, we want to lower the ratio of omega-6 and raise the ratio of omega-3 in the family diet. There are three ways to accomplish this task. Method one would be to learn the arts of hunting and fishing and obtain all meats from the wild. The second method would be to buy "free range meats" from the health food store. The third, and least expensive method, incorporates supplementation with fish and flax oil. I recommend supplementation with fish and flax oil.

In addition to morning supplementation, we can take these oils whenever we eat meat other than fish. While wild fish contain an abundance of omega-3 fatty acids, the meats we buy in the supermarket contain an abundance of omega-6 fatty acids. Supplementing protein intake

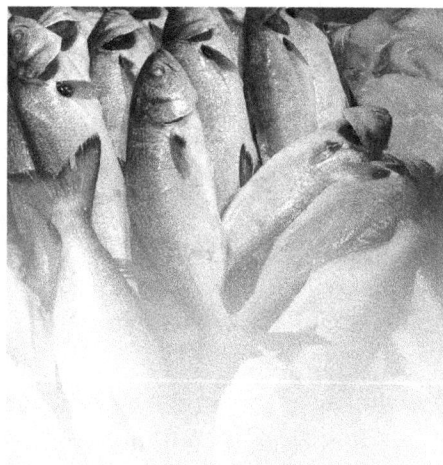

with fish and flax oils mimics the food combination that the hunter/gatherers subsisted on, and helps achieve the healthy 3:1 ratio we desire.

Considering the toxic world we live in, some people will not consume fish oil, canned tuna, or even fish caught in the wild, fearing the possibility of mercury or heavy metal poisoning.

A supplement that we will introduce, glutathione, is a natural substance that the body makes. Glutathione binds to harmful toxins and heavy metals, so that they may be dispelled from the body.

This fact has given me a lot of "peace of mind" in this toxic world in which we live. While there may never be a problem, with the foods and supplements we take into the body, I like the "extra insurance" that glutathione supplementation gives me.

Acidophilus

Acidophilus is friendly bacteria. Believe it or not, bacteria, called intestinal flora, is suppose to be living in the intestines. This flora is important to the immune system for fighting sickness and disease. Medications such as antibiotics easily destroy this fragile flora.

Yogurt is full of probiotic cultures such as acidophilus and Bifidus. If yogurt is something your child will not eat, consider supplementing with acidophilus and/or Bifidus capsules.

Chromium Picolinate

This supplement helps regulate blood sugar. Specifically, it helps insulin efficiency by reducing blood glucose levels. As most everyone knows, the key to regulating blood sugar is the key to diabetes prevention.

"Chromium is a mineral that helps to increase the efficiency of insulin, the hormone that controls blood glucose (blood sugar) levels; Picolinate is an amino acid derivative that allows the body to use chromium much more readily." [35]

Insulin efficiency will also help us burn fat.

"Furthermore, since improving the action of insulin also helps the body to use fat as fuel, chromium Picolinate can help reduce obesity." [36]

Glutathione

As stated earlier, Glutathione helps detoxify the body of harmful metals.

"As a detoxifier of heavy metals and drugs it aids in the treatment of blood and liver disorders." [37]

Glutathione, or GSH, has also been used to treat diabetes and many other diseases.

"Intravenous GSH, with GSH as a sodium salt, has been used to treat chemical or radiation poisoning, as well as to treat diabetes and Parkinson's disease." [38]

While diabetes is a chronic "disorder of carbohydrate metabolism," glutathione, or GSH, is an important part of the body chemistry that transforms carbohydrates into energy.

"It is needed for carbohydrate metabolism, and also appears to exert anti-aging effects, aiding in the breakdown of oxidized fats that may contribute to atherosclerosis." [39]

Glutathione is an essential antioxidant that protects the organs of the body. In particular, glutathione protects the lungs and pancreas. The responsibility of the pancreas is to produce insulin for the body. Thus, in the short-term and the long-term, glutathione is an important supplement for diabetes prevention.

Considering the role glutathione plays in the fight against obesity and its ability to extend both the length and quality of life, I recommend a daily supplement of glutathione for both parent and child.

Weigh the Difference

Example: Glutathioine is an important antioxidant for the human body. Although our bodies make glutathioine, we also obtain trace amounts of it through the raw vegetables we eat. The glutathioine content of one 500 mg capsule is comparable to the same content found in several raw potatoes. Which would you rather eat?

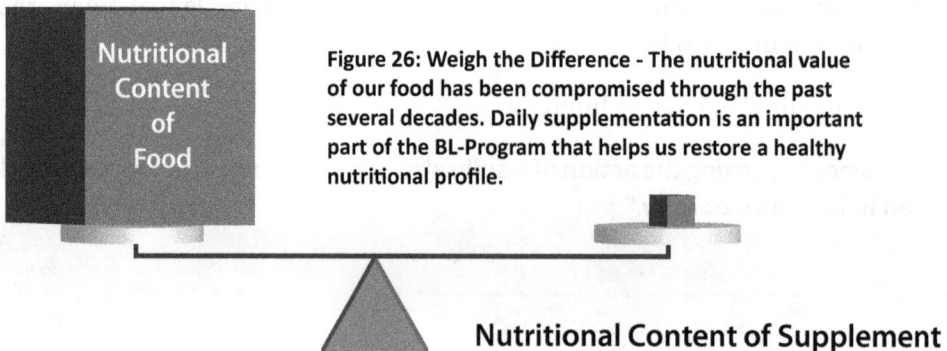

Figure 26: Weigh the Difference - The nutritional value of our food has been compromised through the past several decades. Daily supplementation is an important part of the BL-Program that helps us restore a healthy nutritional profile.

Nutritional Content of Food

Nutritional Content of Supplement

The Elixir of Life

While talking to a health food expert one day, he told me of a man who suffered from many ailments. This man was overweight, chronically fatigued, suffered flu like symptoms and had joint pain. He felt like an old man, even though he was only 45 years old. Over the course of a year, this man tried most everything within the health food store, but to no avail.

The health food expert continued his story by saying that one day this individual with ill health bounced into his shop happy as can be. With a gleam in his eye and conviction in his voice, he told the health food expert, "I have found the elixir of life, glutathione!"

Centuries ago, people known as alchemists searched in vain for the elixir of life, a substance that would give them eternal youth and physical well-being.

The more I learn about glutathione, the more I have come to believe that even though there is no such thing as an elixir of life, glutathione comes closest to making such a claim.

Glutathione - Made Within the Body

Every living thing, including humans, produce glutathione within the cells of their body. It is essential for life! Glutathione is a tripeptide made of three amino acids, glycine, glutamine, and cysteine. These three combine together to detoxify the inner cell of harmful substances.

"Glutathione protects cells in several ways. It neutralizes oxygen molecules before they can harm cells. Together with selenium, it forms the enzyme glutathione peroxidase, which neutralizes hydrogen peroxide." [40]

In the Human Body, Glutathione is an Important Antioxidant

After glutathione performs important functions within the cells of the body, the cells export some glutathione to the blood stream. The blood stream transports glutathione to the lungs and pancreas, and every joint and organ of the body to act as a shield or antioxidant.

"It is a powerful antioxidant that inhibits the formation of, and protects against cellular damage from, free radicals" [41]

GSH thus is an essential antioxidant at the cellular level but also provides important protection at a larger scale, to the organs of the body.

"Glutathione protects not only individual cells but also the tissues of the arteries, brain, heart, immune cells, kidneys, lenses of the eyes, liver, lungs, and skin against oxidant damage." [42]
"GSH provides powerful antioxidant protection to body systems heavily exposed to reactive oxygen species, such as the lung." [43]

Most people have heard the term antioxidant, but do not know what an antioxidant does, and why they are an important part of human vitality. The following picture **(Figure 27)** is a symbolic representation of how glutathione works as an antioxidant.

Your body's immune system uses certain substances to fight and kill germs. Among these germ-fighting substances are oxidants, elastase, and certain free radicals, symbolized in this picture by bullets and acid.

"Free radicals produced by the immune system destroy viruses and bacteria." [44]

As the immune system unleashes these substances to kill harmful germs, the organs of the body need to be protected from this same ammunition. To protect the organs of the body from its own immune system, antioxidants act as the shield.

"By destroying free radicals, antioxidants help detoxify and protect the body." [45]

This diagram **(Figure 27)** shows how the immune system's ammunition of oxidants and elastase kills germs while glutathione stands between the lungs/pancreas or other organs of the body, giving protection.

Glutathione as an Antioxidant

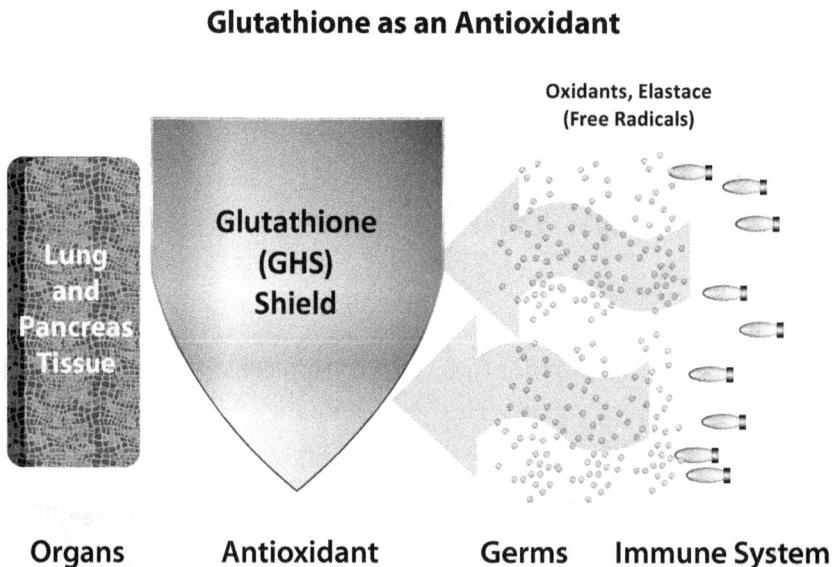

Organs   Antioxidant   Germs   Immune System

Figure 27: Glutathione as an Antioxidant - Glutathione acts as a shield to protect the joints and organs of the body from the harmful effects of the immune system.

With this basic understanding of glutathione, we can begin to appreciate why it may be considered the elixir of life. Research shows that the average male makes approximately 10 grams of glutathione a day. Research also shows that the amount of glutathione produced by the body drops off after the age of 40.

"As we age, glutathione levels decline." [46]

The next visual **(Figure 28)**, represents what happens to the glutathione shield, as we get older. With the body producing less glutathione, the GSH shield diminishes, allowing oxidant damage to the organs and joints of the body.

While the deterioration caused by the reduction of glutathione is imperceptible at the age of 40, we can see the long-term consequences in the body at 60 or 80 years of age. Consequences of oxidant damage include wrinkles, arthritis, and weakening of the organs of the body.

Glutathione as Healer

There are many other relevant processes in the human body to which glutathione plays an essential role.

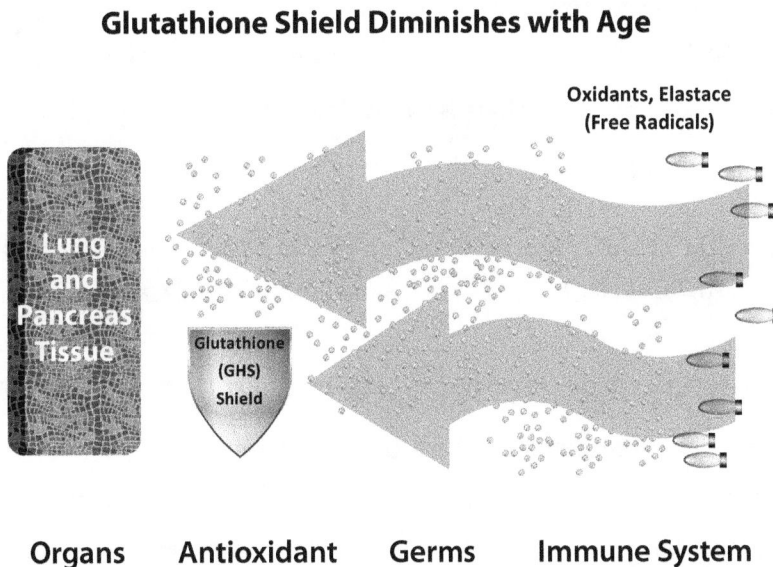

Glutathione Shield Diminishes with Age

Figure 28: Glutathione Shield Diminishes with Age - Our body's ability to make glutathione diminishes after the age of 40. Oxidant damage caused by the breakdown of the GHS shield, is a big factor in the aging process.

In terms of weight management, glutathione is probably better described as an important part of body chemistry that helps us achieve "ideal weight." While it plays an important role in diabetes prevention and the weight gain often associated with that disease, glutathione also helps patients who need to gain weight.

People with the genetic disease cystic fibrosis have trouble gaining weight. The reason these patients cannot gain weight has to do with the pathways that carry digestive enzymes to the intestines. People with this disease have thick sticky mucus that block the digestive enzyme pathways. Glutathione is one of the main mucus-cleaving agents of the body. Supplementation of glutathione by CF patients, breaks up the mucus that typically blocks enzyme pathways, thereby allowing patients with this disease to gain weight.

"Because of its chemistry, GSH, like N-Acetylcysteine (NAC), is able to cleave disulfide bonds, which serves to reduce the viscoelasticity of mucus when the glutathione system is functioning normally." [47]

I know three young brothers that have cystic fibrosis. They each take a daily oral supplementation of glutathione. Comparing their weight and height to normal children without cystic fibrosis, these three brothers fall within the 95th, 75th, and 50th percent brackets for their age group. This is remarkable! Compared to normal children, children with CF typically fall below the 25th percent bracket for their age group.

Glutathione plays an essential role in the body's overall immune system. It acts as a regulator and trigger for the inflammation process.

"A third property of reduced glutathione is to regulate inflammation and immune response." [48]

One only needs to consider the many diseases where glutathione helps the ailing patient, to appreciate this elixir of life. These include but are not limited to; arthritis, macular degeneration, cystic fibrosis, emphysema, cirrhosis of the liver, diabetes, colitis, heavy metal poisoning, AIDS, autism.

Glutathione as a Practical Supplement

People are not taking advantage of glutathione supplementation, believing that GSH is not absorbed into the blood, when taken orally. Recent research has proven otherwise.

"Fortunately, the number and sophistication of recent research articles demonstrating that GSH is taken up intact from the small intestine outweigh those denying that such uptake occurs." [49]

As one who suffered from arthritis, oral glutathione has worked for me. It has made a huge difference in the quality of my life. I am virtually pain free and my joints exhibit normal mobility. I know this happened because oral glutathione worked. GSH was getting to my joints.

Another factor inhibiting some people from supplementing with glutathione is the cost. The way that some people get around this issue is to supplement with cysteine, which promotes the making of glutathione in the cells. However we recommend that your child does not use this method for two reasons. Overdosing with cysteine can be toxic. Secondly, there is evidence that cysteine alone can cause problems with those who are prone to diabetes.

"People who have diabetes should be cautious about taking supplemental cysteine because it is capable of inactivating insulin." [50]

My family has supplemented with glutathione for several years. GHS has reduced the amount of colds and flu in the home. While we have never used it for radiation poisoning, topically we have mixed glutathione with olive oil to get rid of toxins caused by spider bites and stings from bees. It is a very practical supplement for the long-term and short-term.

Considering all the health benefits that glutathione supplementation offers, it is well worth the investment. The philosophy that I use concerning glutathione cost is like the philosophy behind buying oil for my car, or the philosophy behind the Bases Loaded Program itself. Preventing a fire from happening, is better than paying for fire damage.

Oil for the Car = Glutathione for the Body

How important is glutathione to the body? Let us once again compare the human body to an automobile. If the food and water we put in the body is comparable to the fuel and water needed to make a car run, than glutathione would be comparable to the oil of the car. The oil "protects" the vital parts of an engine from heat, wear and tear. Without oil, a car would eventually stop running. So it is with the body. Without glutathione, we would stop running!

When to take Supplements

Be sure to read labels and consult with health food experts as to the proper daily dosage for all of the supplements that your family chooses to take. The amount for your child will be different from the amount an adult takes. Wash all your supplements down with a little orange juice for some extra vitamin C.

Since supplements are nutrients that are suppose to be in food, let us take them after breakfast. Maybe we can fool the body into believing that we are at grandmother's house back in the 1950's, having dinner.

When it comes to fish and flax oil as stated earlier, feel free to supplement whenever eating meat other than fish, to mimic the protein and good fat that the hunter/gatherers had in their diet.

Now all these memories of Grandma's house and her dinners have made me hungry. I am going to grab a healthy snack! Please grab a healthy snack too and meet me back here. The next chapter contains a truly significant puzzle piece in the construction of the childhood obesity puzzle! Your family will not want to miss it!

Protein Antioxidant Shake

Here is an example of combining good foods and powerful supplements into a healthy snack. Combine the following ingredients into a blender, mix up, and serve on a hot summer's day!

- **Two cups 1% milk**

- **A few cubes of ice**

- **Couple Tablespoons plain yogurt**

- **One frozen banana**

- **Half of an avocado**

- **500 mg glutathione**

- **Scoop of powder protein supplement**

- **Agave syrup and vanilla extract to taste.**

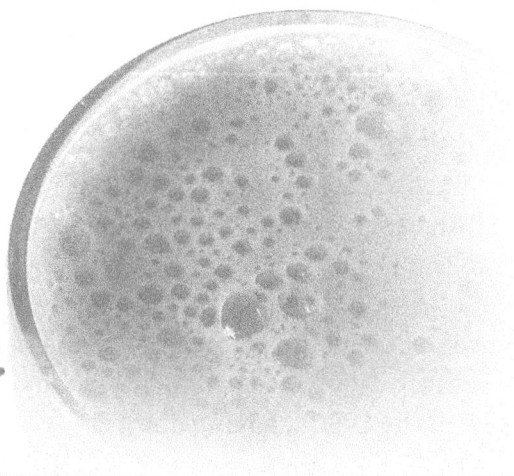

Check Your Understanding

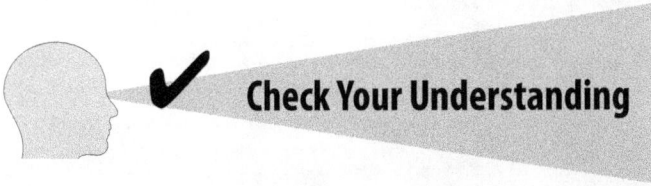

1. **Why has the nutritional profile of food diminished in recent decades?**

    Answer: *The nutritional profile of food has diminished due to fertilization practices and depletion of nutrients from the soil. Food processing has also added to this problem.*

2. **How does supplementation reduce cravings and fight childhood obesity?**

    Answer: *When nutrients are missing from food, strong cravings occur in the human body, which often cause a person to overeat. Supplementation helps to satisfy the nutritional needs of the body and, therefore, prevent cravings. Supplementation thus fights obesity by reducing the tendency to overeat.*

3. **Which supplements help insulin efficiency and carbohydrate metabolism?**

    Answer: *Chromium Picolinate and glutathione help insulin efficiency and carbohydrate metabolism.*

4. **Which supplement promotes intestinal flora?**

    Answer: *Acidophilus/Bifidus promotes friendly bacteria.*

5. **Which supplements will improve the ratio of omega-3 within the family diet?**

    Answer: *Fish oil and flax oil improve the ratio of omega-3 fatty acids that we desire.*

6. **What powerful antioxidant is sometimes called "the elixir of life?"**

    Answer: *Glutathione is sometimes called the elixir of life.*

7. **What are the harmful substances deflected by the human body's glutathione shield?**

    Answer: *Glutathione shields the organs of the human body from oxidants and the harmful ammunition of the immune system.*

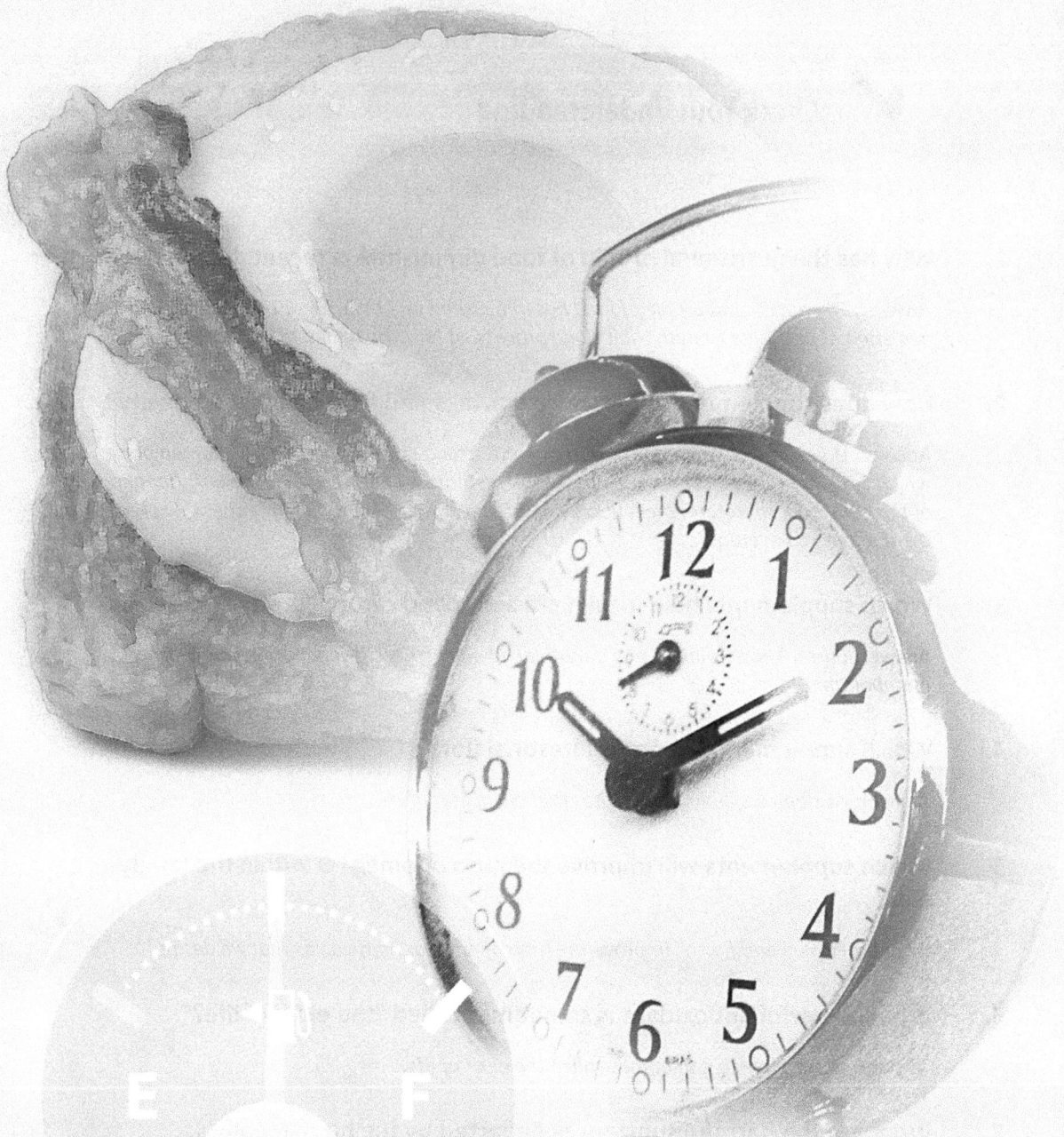

The key to understanding childhood obesity is to understand metabolism's fuel gauge.

Fasting

Chapter

10

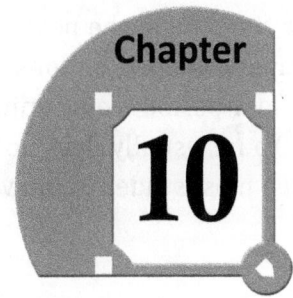

We have discussed Bases Loaded from the perspective of "when to eat." Now let us view it from the perspective of when not to eat. "Fasting," the very word brings fear to the heart of all who have ever dieted. Let your mind, not worry, for this chapter will teach the concept of proper fasting. The word "fasting" means to do without food or drink or both for an extended period. Believe it or not, every normal adult fasts once a day.

This fast lasts for at least eight hours, or one third of a 24-hour day. Unless one has mastered the art of eating and drinking while unconscious, then a fast occurs while sleeping. The definition of the term "breakfast," derives from the above concept. When we eat the first food of the day after waking, we literally break the fast. The fact that fasting is a natural daily phenomenon can make us all feel better about this scary subject. Some people with medical conditions should only fast during the hours that they sleep. Be sure to heed your doctor's advice concerning these matters. Most human beings, though, fast for longer than 8 hours per day. Most people do not feel hungry until about 12-hours after they eat the last food of the evening. This means that most people spend half of a twenty-four hour day in a state of fasting.

Improper Fasting

It does not seem that we go without eating for half the day. If we consider recent research, as well as one's own experiences, we might be surprised when we start adding up the hours.

"Research shows that people who have dinner late in the evening are more likely to skip breakfast the following morning." [51]

Some of us like to eat food right up until we go to sleep. We go to bed at midnight, get up early, and then rush out the door to go to work. Perhaps we have some coffee or juice, but food in the morning is not that appealing. Could it be that the body has a natural capacity or need to fast?

"By relieving the body of the work of digesting foods, fasting permits the system to rid itself of toxins while facilitating healing." ... **"By fasting regularly, you give all of your organs a rest, and thus help reverse the aging process and live a longer and healthier life."** [52]

The timeline in the next visual **(Figure 29)** depicts the 12-hour fast cycle for most people in the developed nations of the world. Most children go to bed before midnight and the 12-hour period would adjust accordingly. A person who snacks till midnight and wakes at 8:00 a.m., usually does not feel hungry again till 11:00 a.m., or noon. Conveniently, this is when most students and working people eat lunch.

Fasting in the Fast Lane
(Improper Fasting)

4 p.m.	8 p.m.	Sleep Fasting—No Food	Wake Little to no food	12 Noon	4 p.m.
		12 Midnight	8 a.m.		

Figure 29: Fasting in the Fast Lane or Improper Fasting - The daily fasting cycle for most people in developed nations roughly spans the 12 hours from midnight to noon.

Natural Sunset Cycle

The next timeline **(Figure 30)** depicts the 12-hour fast cycle advocated by the Bases Loaded Program. I refer to this time, from sunset to sunrise as the "Natural Sunset Cycle" (NS-Cycle), and the time from sunrise to sunset as the "Natural Eating Cycle" (NE-Cycle). We do not have to go too far back in American history to find that the vast majority of people followed these natural cycles. The daylight hours were the hours that great-great grandparents worked and ate. Dinner, the last meal of the day, coincided with sunset and signified the end of food consumption. The BL-Plan thus represents a return to the natural cycles of eating and refraining from food (sun setting on food) that they practiced. It represents a return to working with the metabolism instead of against it.

Going further back into history we find that the natural cycle of eating was, for the most part, practiced by the hunter/gatherers. It probably was not the preferred way of eating. The preferred way was dependent upon a successful hunt. Since obtaining food was the main focus of life for the hunter/gatherers, a successful hunt was most likely celebrated with a feast that extended into the late evening. Most likely, these celebrations were ritualistic but had a practical purpose too. Meat spoils quickly in warm climates. This fact required the hunter/gatherer tribe to eat continuously until the animal was totally consumed.

Fasting in the Slow Lane
(Natural Sunset Cycle)

4 p.m.	Little to no food	Sleep Fasting—No Food	8 a.m.	12 Noon	4 p.m.
4 p.m.	8 p.m.	12 Midnight	8 a.m.	12 Noon	4 p.m.

Figure 30: Fasting in the Slow Lane or Natural Sunset Cycle - The daily fasting cycle advocated by the BL-Program roughly spans the 12 hours from 8 p.m. to 8 a.m.

Since successful hunting was sporadic at best, the hunter/gatherers spent most days eating rationed gathered items. They would go to sleep early so that they might awake early and try their luck at hunting again. When one thinks about it, modern society has placed human beings into a very unnatural position. School and work schedules have taken top priority in the hectic developed world that we live. We are on the "Saturday Morning Method" of starting the day. We choose to delay food until we get all those necessary morning chores done. We still eat in a 12-hour cycle, but instead of eating from sunrise to sunset, we tend to eat from noon till midnight. This simple four hour shift has caused great havoc for the metabolism and presents itself as a major contributor to the modern day obesity epidemic.

"A study published in the American Journal of Epidemiology reported that those who miss breakfast are 4½ times more likely to be obese than those who eat a morning meal. [53]

There are more contributing factors to the obesity dilemma that we will consider later. For now, let us focus on how modern man has tried to deal with the weight gain that has occurred, in large measure, because of ignorance concerning these cycles.

Dieting

What is dieting? Sometimes a doctor will prescribe certain dietary restrictions to a patient due to a particular medical condition. It goes without saying that a patient should heed the advice of their doctor concerning their particular medical condition. This situation is not the common definition of dieting.

The definition of dieting that most Americans identify with, is a situation where a person makes a conscious choice, to reduce the amount of calories or types of food that they consume, in the course of a day in order to lose weight. Along with this limitation of food intake, dieting usually involves an exercise program.

Within the context of the above definition, we find many varieties of diet programs. There are some programs that cut out the intake of carbohydrates, others that cut out proteins. Many modern diets have reduced the amount of fat intake without distinguishing good fats from bad fats. Some diets allow us to eat whatever we want but restrict us to a specific amount of calories. Some diets cut out the junk food and cut the amount of calories we consume. Extreme diets reduce the amount of calories to starvation levels and limit the types of foods we can eat.

With these thoughts concerning dieting in mind, let us consider the Bases Loaded understanding of dieting.

As reflected in the next visual **(Figure 31)** we consider dieting, in the general sense of the word, to be a form of improper fasting. From my perspective, limiting calories, or limiting nutritional variety during the twelve hour natural eating cycle constitutes improper fasting. Now let us pause a moment and consider the big picture from the Bases Loaded perspective. One of the biggest contributing factors of childhood obesity, and obesity for all ages is the practice of improper fasting. It seems logical that the first step to undo the damage caused by improper fasting, is to put back into one's life the natural 12-hour eating cycle that works best with metabolism. Instead of taking this logical step, Americans have tried to undo the negative effects of improper fasting using more improper fasting!

Dieting
(Improper Fasting)

Little to no food		Sleep Fasting—No Food	Little to no food		
4 p.m.	8 p.m.	12 Midnight	8 a.m.	12 Noon	4 p.m.

Figure 31: Dieting or Improper Fasting - Dieting is essentially a non-stop fast where the body is receiving little to no food, 24 hours a day.

Common sense tells us that if we try to solve a problem with more of the same problem that it will only compound the problem. That is certainly the case when we consider the realm of dieting and its effect on metabolism. Ironically, dieting puts the dieter into starvation mode, the very condition that the hunter/gathers wanted to avoid. The reason dieting fails in a general sense has to do with the fact that we in the developed world have food all around us. Dieters put themselves in a tortuous situation where they deprive themselves of food while the food is easily within their reach. Eventually instincts take over, and cravings compel the dieter to eat, and make up for lost time.

Dieting and Metabolism's Memory

As we take a more detailed look at dieting, we will come across a small but powerful "missing" puzzle piece. The missing piece has to do with metabolism's memory. Keep in mind that Mr. Metabolism is a very old man. Like many of us as we age, Mr. Metabolism has a sharp long-term memory. On the other hand, his short-term memory is not as good as a younger person.

Read these next sections carefully, for they will help your understanding of the phenomenon of childhood obesity in a new way!

Metabolism's Long-Term Memory

We have already encountered Mr. Metabolism's long-term memory earlier in the book. Let us review.

"If you starve your body of certain nutrients the next time you introduce it, your body will store it, which is what the body does in time of famine." [54]

In other words, diets that advocate the cutting out of certain nutrients like carbohydrates, or proteins, fight against metabolism's long-term memory. The metabolism interprets these deficiencies as periods of famine or meat scarcity. Mr. Metabolism stores the memory of a deficiency and will not forget it.

It does not matter how much time passes, if it is several days, weeks, or months, metabolism will hold on to this piece of memory. Not only does the metabolism hold onto this memory, it will create strong cravings within the body to motivate us to fill the nutritional void. The body takes upon itself what I call "partial starvation mode." As we discussed earlier, people try to fill the nutritional void caused by "partial starvation mode" in different ways. The non-dieter often fills the void using junk food. The dieter will fill the void by purposely consuming types of food that are different from the nutrient that the body is craving. These situations initially lead to overeating and unwanted weight gain.

Once the dieter starts eating the deficient nutrient, again, they face another challenge. They compulsively eat the craved food. The metabolism inspires an "over" eating of the lost nutrient. The metabolism ships the extra fuel to fat storage, to be used in case the "perceived famine" were to extend into the days and weeks ahead. Instead of solving the original problem, this "overeating," thus compounds the original weight gain problem.

Metabolism's Short-Term or Limited Memory

It may seem from the explanation above that metabolism's memory is perfect. I believe that when it comes to nutritional deficiencies, the metabolism is perfect. It has a memory that cannot be fooled. When it comes to the other aspect of conventional dieting, that of calorie intake, I think the metabolism is easily fooled.

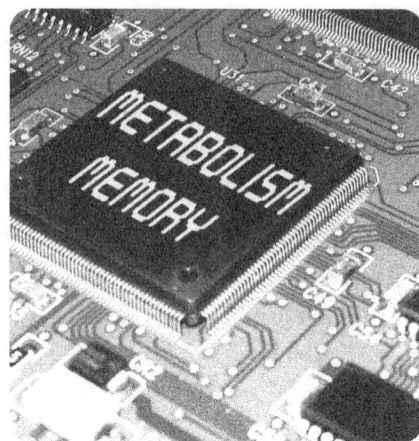

In my opinion, when it comes to calories, Mr. Metabolism has a particularly poor, short-term memory. Metabolism has a "limited memory" that only extends back as far as when it awoke from a good night's sleep. In other words, well rested metabolism cannot remember the calorie intake from the previous day. It erases memory! Each day is a new beginning, a new creation for the metabolism.

If this theory of "limited memory" is correct, then what we have here is truly important indeed! With this information, not only will we be able to explain the folly of conventional dieting, but we will have all the pieces we need to complete the childhood obesity puzzle!

Metabolism's Fuel Gauge

We can compare metabolism's limited memory of calorie intake, to a fuel gauge on a car **(Figure 32)**. Notice that a fuel gauge divides fuel into sections. The top section designates a full tank of fuel. A large line in the middle designates a half tank of fuel.

The bottom section designates a near empty, and an empty tank. Sometimes we refer to the fuel within the bottom one eighth section as reserve fuel.

Newer cars have little alarms and lights to let the driver know that their fuel is at this reserve level and is about to run out. When a driver hears this fuel alarm, they immediately look down to their dashboard and notice that the fuel gauge is near the E. How much reserve fuel is in the tank and how far can a driver go before their car runs out of fuel? Some people know the answers to these questions with their own car.

I do not know the answers for my own car. Sure, I know that my car gets so many miles to the gallon, and I guess that I have one, maybe two gallons of fuel left, so I hurry myself to

Metabolism's Fuel Gauge

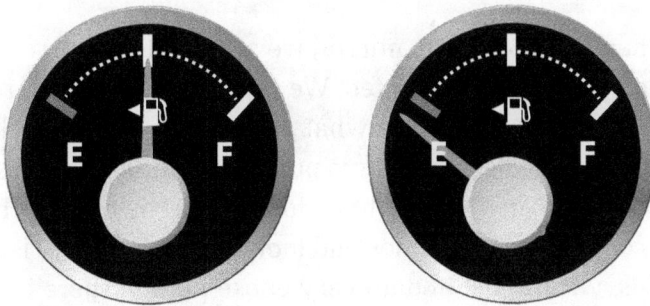

Figure 32: Metabolism's Fuel Gauge - Metabolism has a "limited memory" which can be compared to the reserve tank and alarm system of a fuel gauge.

the nearest fuel station to avoid the awful situation of running out of gas with a car full of energetic children!

How does this situation compare to metabolism's short-term memory? The E on metabolism's fuel gauge represents the awful situation of starvation. The reserve tank, with all its buzzers and lights sound their alarm to one's metabolism every morning, as soon as the body gets out of bed. That is right! When we awake from fasting, whether we have fasted for 8 hours or 12 hours, the fuel gauge is almost on E, and the alarms tell metabolism that the body needs fuel quickly because it is now running on reserve. What is the amount of fuel left in the tank? That is different for each person.

The reserve energy tanks of the human body, as mentioned earlier, are the fat cells of the body. For some people, this amount of energy weighs 2 pounds, for others it is 20 pounds or 200 pounds. Because of metabolism's limited memory concerning calorie intake, it does not know how much energy is in storage. Whether it is 2 pounds or 200 pounds, metabolism can only guess that it has one or two pounds left before energy runs out and the process of starvation begins.

Mr. Metabolism faces another question. He does not know how far it is to the next fuel station. Is it one mile or one hundred miles to the next station? Will this reserve tank supply the body's energy needs for the next day, ten days, or month?

It is this uncertainty on Mr. Metabolism's part, which creates a huge irony in the battle with obesity. Because of Mr. Metabolism's uncertainty concerning fuel amount and expenditure distance, he does what every cautious driver does in the same situation. He slows way down to conserve fuel. In Mr. Metabolism's language, he slows down to starvation mode.

Obesity's Paradox

See the paradox? When we look in the mirror, we see what all the rest of the world sees. We see a person who appears to be well fed. We chastise ourselves for being overweight. Children also look in the mirror and see what all the rest of the world sees. They see a person who appears to be overfed, but this is putting it kindly. A child's world is different from an adult's world. When an overweight child looks in the mirror, they also remember all the fat jokes, the condescending names and looks given them by classmates. The irony of the situation is this; within just about every obese person there is another extremely skinny person. That person is Mr. Metabolism. He is skinny because he truly believes that the body is starving! Mr. Metabolism is blind to the extra fuel tanks that we carry around with us. When metabolism believes we are starving, it makes sure that we feel all the symptoms of starvation. Even if, we carry 40 lbs of reserve fuel, we will feel hungry and tired. It will seem that we have no energy. We are grumpy all day long and why not? It is hard for us to feel happy when we feel we are starving. Compounding these physical feelings are the psychological issues, the emotional stress we feel as we view ourselves in the mirror. We begin to believe that, in certain respects, we are failures.

Herein we find the missing puzzle piece of childhood obesity! The key to understanding childhood obesity, is to understand metabolism's fuel gauge, and how this anciently programmed instrument is being deceived in the context of today's modern lifestyle.

More on Metabolism's Limited Memory

One might ask, "How come metabolism's fuel gauge does not know exactly how much reserve fuel is on hand?"

The hunter/gatherer faced day-to-day survival as the given reality. It is hard for us to imagine a life where starvation, or death from a predator, is a daily concern. Metabolism is designed with these two daily threats in mind.

Because the food was scarce, the hunter/gatherers' metabolism operated in starvation mode most of the time. Metabolism's main task was to conserve every particle of energy, letting nothing go to waste. Even the regulation process could not waste energy.

Seen in this light, metabolism's memory, or fuel gauge, is a highly efficient way to handle the problem. To program metabolism in such a way that it had to continually inventory a reserve of fuel that was seldom there would have been a waste of energy. Conserving energy, no matter how small that energy was, meant the difference between life and death for the species.

Starvation mode had another long-range objective for the species. Since the hunter/ gatherers spent much of their time feeling hungry, it forced them to take a more humble approach to life than the swift and strong animal predators around them. Instead of using their speed or strength, to prevail, human ancestors used their brains. Seen in this light, metabolism's programming played a critical role in the advancement of the human species.

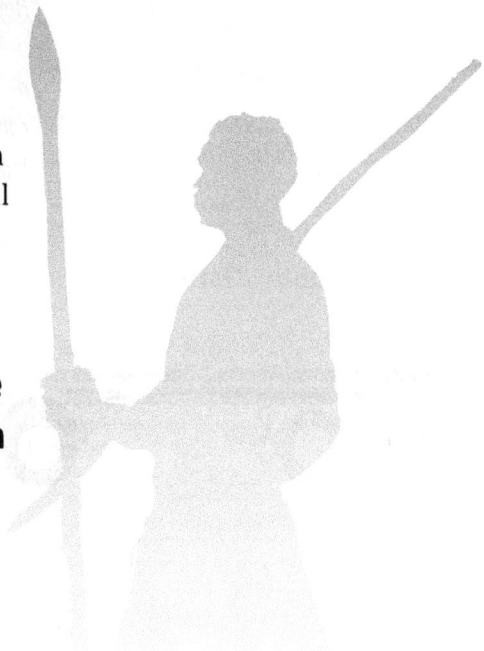

It is hard for us to imagine a life where starvation or death from a predator, is a daily concern. Metabolism is designed with these two daily threats in mind.

The Parable of the Wise Businessman

We can compare metabolism, and its memory, to a bank account, set up for a business that was struggling to survive. The businessman set up the business during hard times. The businessman had to decide what account he wanted for his business. Was it to be a deluxe bank account or a low activity bank account? The low activity account was not as fancy as the deluxe account, but it was seven dollars a month cheaper than the deluxe account. The businessman wisely chose the low activity account. He reasoned that although seven dollars amounted to very little money, still every little bit counted for his struggling business.

We can compare the metabolism's short-term memory to the low activity account. It does not need as much energy to work as a complicated system. It protects and warns us concerning available assets, without having to continually inventory the amount in reserve.

Metabolism's "Limited Memory"

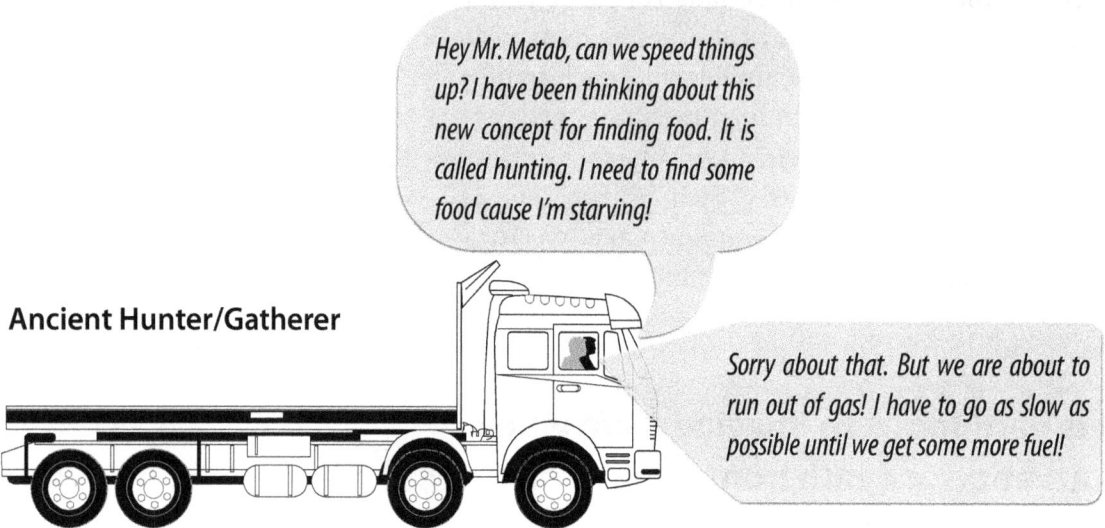

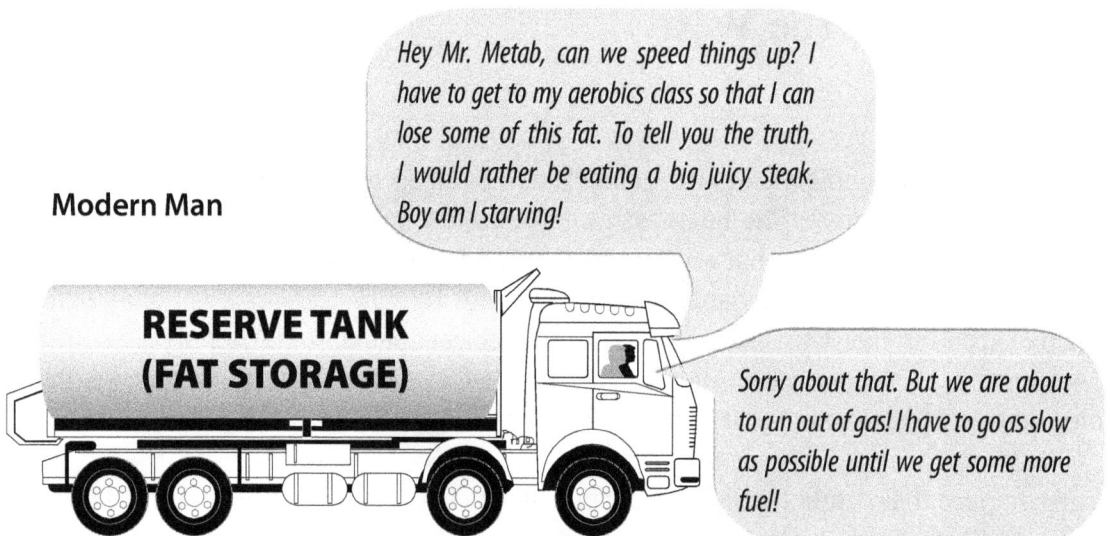

Figure 33: Metabolism's Limited Memory - Metabolism has a poor short-term memory. It cannot remember the caloric intake from the previous day, or how much fuel is in fat storage. Metabolism responds to fasting in the morning hours by slowing down, to conserve energy, regardless of the amount of fuel in fat storage.

✔ Check Your Understanding

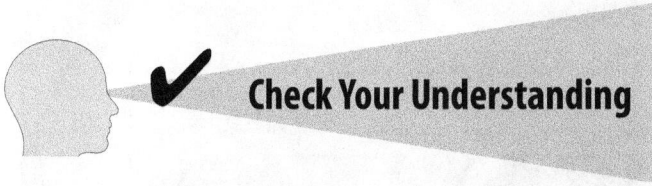

1. **Is it true that people tend to eat in eight-hour cycles?**

   Answer: *False, most people eat and fast in alternating twelve hour cycles.*

2. **According to the BL-Program, what is the Natural Sunset Cycle?**

   Answer: *It refers to refraining from food during the twelve hours between sunset and sunrise.*

3. **Describe Mr. Metabolism's long-term memory.**

   Answer: *Metabolism will remember any deficient nutrient the body is missing, no matter how much time has elapsed from the time the nutrient was last consumed by the body.*

4. **Describe Mr. Metabolism's short-term memory.**

   Answer: *Metabolism erases memory during sleep so that it forgets calorie intake from the previous day, and all fat storage.*

5. **To what can we compare metabolism's limited memory?**

   Answer: *Metabolism's limited memory can be compared to the fuel gauge of a car.*

6. **List the similarities of the images in Figure 33.**

   Answer: *Both vehicles are the same basic make/model. Both vehicles are traveling slow. Both men feel starved. In both images, Mr. Metab thinks fuel is low. He is not aware of how much fuel is actually in the reserve tank.*

7. **List the differences between the two images in Figure 33.**

   Answer: *The amount of fuel in the reserve tanks are different, making the modern vehicle appear larger. The amount of reserve fuel weighs down the modern vehicle. Modern man is very aware of the size of his reserve storage tank while this is not so with the hunter/gatherer. Starvation mode is motivating the hunter/gatherer to new discoveries while the modern man preoccupies himself with thoughts of his reserve storage tank, as well as the feelings of hunger that he feels.*

8. **Modern man, like the hunter/gatherer, feels starved even though he carries plenty of reserve fuel. Explain this paradox?**

   Answer: *Modern man feels starved because metabolism believes the body is starving. Ignorance of the large quantity of readily available fat reserves can only be explained by the notion that metabolism has forgotten about them. Metabolism has a limited memory.*

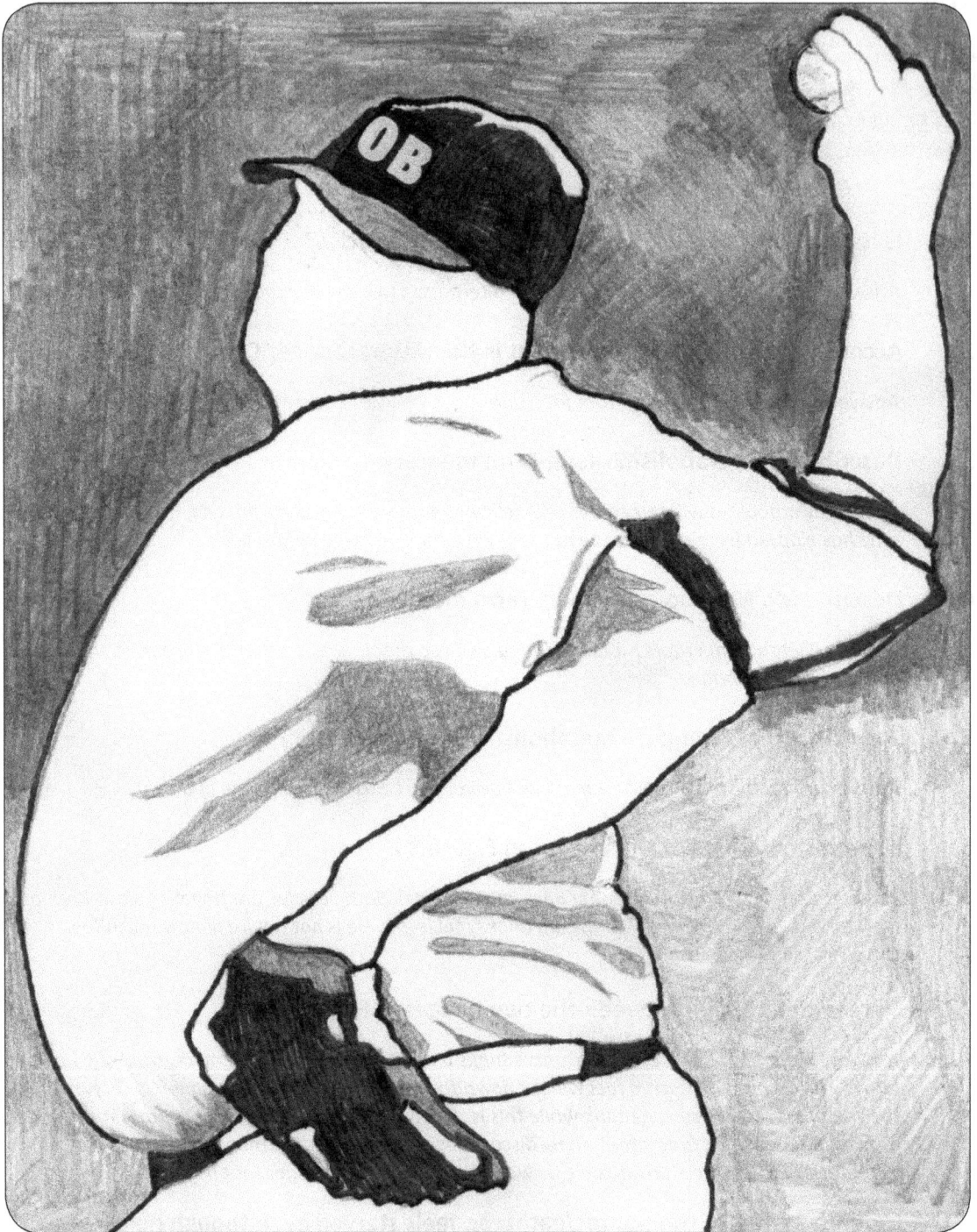

Obesity wants us to be in starvation mode 24 hours a day!

Obesity's Three Pitches

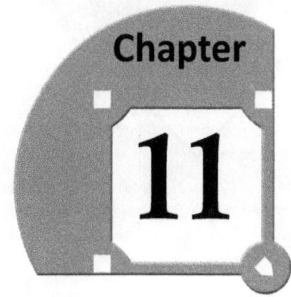

Obesity's Three Daily Baseball Pitches

In baseball terms, we can compare the deception of metabolism's "limited memory," as "Obesity's Three Daily Pitches." Remember Rookie, the child up to bat against the pitcher Obesity? At what three pitches did Rookie strike? They were a fastball, curveball, and changeup pitch in that order.

We can compare Obesity's fastball to "fasting" in the morning. We can compare Obesity's curveball to the deception that occurs from metabolism's limited memory. We can also compare the emotional and psychological stress that plays out in the lives of those who fast improperly as Obesity's "changeup pitch."

Just like a professional pitcher, Obesity uses a fastball to set up the next two deceptive pitches, tricking the batter to expect a certain type of pitch, but delivering something much different.

Using Metabolism's Limited Memory to an Advantage

Now that, we understand this daily deception, we need not be fooled by it. Indeed, understanding this deception allows us to turn things around. How can we use this knowledge to an advantage? The Bases Loaded Program avoids Obesity's pitches of deception. By "breaking" the fast each and every morning that we awake, we avoid starvation mode, Obesity's curveball. By satisfying hunger, getting the bulk of food during the day, we avoid the feelings of starvation that intensify the emotional and psychological stress of being overweight. We avoid Obesity's changeup pitch.

The program not only avoids these pitches of deception it throws them back to Obesity. By organizing the evenings with physical activity, we deceive the metabolism in a good way. Remember, the metabolism has no understanding of exercise or the concept of having fun. It believes that physical activity is the body's attempt to find food. In the Bases Loaded Program, we provide fuel for Mr. Metabolism all day, so he does not believe the body is

OBESITY

—

Fastballs
Curveballs
Change-ups

CATCHER
Discouragement
Hopelessness
Failure

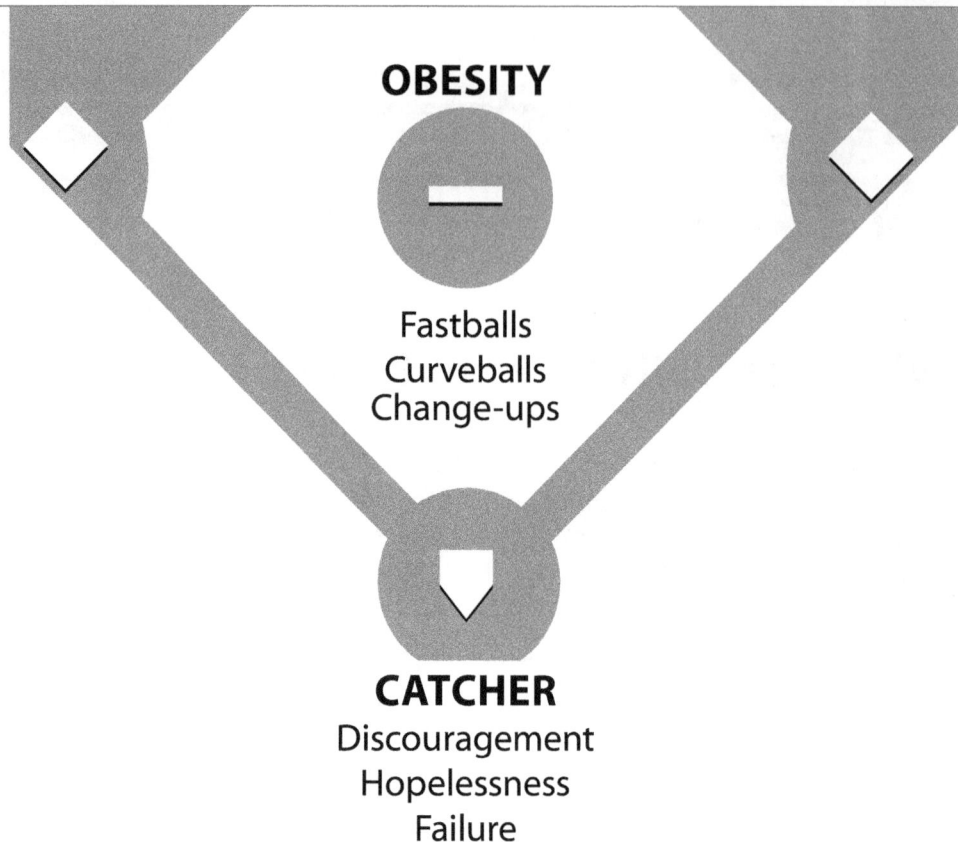

starving. At night, Mr. Metabolism would like to start getting ready for sleep, but since we have been good to him during the day, he is willing to work with us and deliver the energy needed for that last hunt (workout) of the evening.

After a workout, we send Mr. Metabolism to bed without his anticipated midnight snack. Do not feel bad about having fooled him. At this time of the evening, metabolism prefers sleep to food. After a well rested night, Mr. Metabolism will awake and not remember a thing. Just remember to use the "Sweet Old Visiting Grandma Method" with him in the morning, to wake him and satisfy his hunger, and he will provide the energy needs for another great day.

Is this not a better way to live life? In the introduction of this book, we recounted how Joe described the first few weeks of his program in positive terms. He said; "I feel better," and "This is awesome." He felt this way not because he had lost a bunch of weight. Rather, he felt free from the shackles of deception that had him bound. Eating a good breakfast, and eating the bulk of his food during the day allowed Joe to avoid Obesity's deceptive pitches. He no longer felt starved. Joe suddenly had the energy to do things. With the strength and energy to live life, came a feeling of well-being. With the inward physical change came a feeling of rightness in his heart and an inward emotional change. The passing days of Joe's program turned into weeks. With each passing week, feelings of despair began to be replaced with feelings of hope and confidence!

More on Obesity's Three Daily Baseball Pitches

Ever looked close at the arms of a major league pitcher? Compare the throwing arm of a pitcher to his catching arm or glove arm. Do not be surprised to find that the pitching arm is almost twice as big as the catching arm. Over the course of his lifetime, a major league pitcher has thrown uncountable baseballs, making his pitching arm disproportional in size and strength. This strength allows some to throw fastballs in the 90-100 mph range. A pitcher desires to develop a good fastball for two main reasons. First, it is extremely difficult to hit a ball traveling 90-100 mph. In order for a batter to hit a ball traveling that fast, they have to commit to swinging their bat within a second after the pitcher releases the pitch. This brings us to the second reason that a pitcher desires a good fastball.

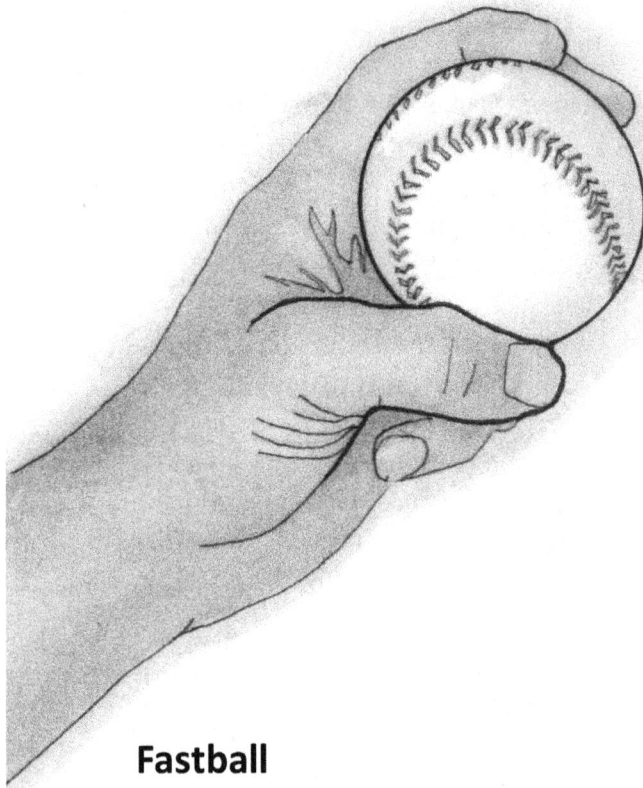

Fastball

A pitcher can use his fastball to manipulate the batter. If the pitcher throws his fastball first in a series of pitches, he can vary the tempo of the next pitches and thus keep the batter guessing as to the speed of the next pitch. This principle works in reverse, as well. When thrown second or third in a series of pitches, a fastball will throw the batter off guard, coming faster to the plate than expected.

A good fastball thus allows the pitcher to control and manipulate the batter. It sends the signal, "I am the boss here!"

Obesity's fastball, "improper fasting," sends the same signal. Whenever we fail to consume the bulk of the daily food in the early part of the day, or intentionally reduce the amount of calories we consume during the day, we allow the pitcher "Obesity" to take charge of the day. We allow Obesity to be the boss, and allow him to pick the tempo of the day.

Guess what pace Obesity will choose for metabolism? Obesity wants the metabolism to be slow! Having successfully delivered his fastball early in the day, Obesity sets us up for a pitch of deception; a curveball.

A curveball is a particularly hard pitch to hit. Some pitchers are able to put a spin on the ball, such that the laces of the ball disrupt the airflow around the ball in its path towards the plate, causing the ball to drop.

When a batter faces a curveball, it appears that the pitcher throws the ball for the strike zone. In a split second, the batter commits to swinging the bat. By the time the ball reaches the plate, it has moved out of position and the batter swings at air. The reality of the event, and the batter's perception of reality were not one in the same.

Curveball

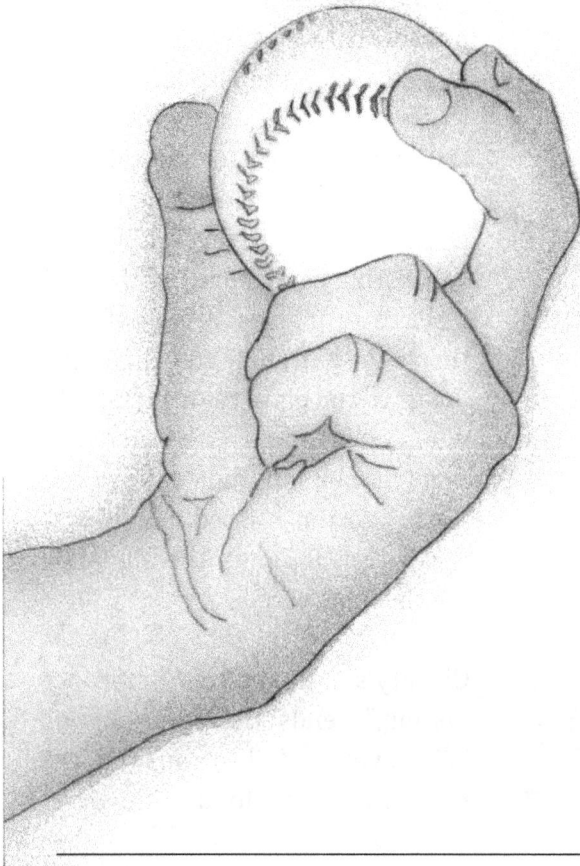

This is exactly the context we experience, once we have struck at Obesity's fastball. Obesity then throws us a curve. The mind knows the reality of the situation; "I had a huge meal before going to bed. I am not starving!" The metabolism, having "limited memory" is fooled by the deception. Starvation mode occurred during the night. The body eats little to no food in the morning, and metabolism cannot remember last night's meal.

Metabolism believes the body is starving and sends the body into starvation mode. Metabolism also gives the body all the symptoms of starvation.

These physical "symptoms of starvation," set us up for Obesity's last pitch. It is a pitch designed to strike us out. If we are not careful, this last pitch will convince us to quit the game.

The changeup pitch is a very effective pitch used to strike out a batter. Remember from the introduction how Rookie swung at the first two pitches, a fastball and a curveball. Obesity threw these two pitches with great speed. A pitcher will sometimes throw the timing of the batter off by following a few fast pitches with a slow pitch, or a changeup pitch. The speed of the ball tricks the batter into swinging before the pitch crosses the plate.

In Obesity's game, the changeup pitch amounts to the emotional and psychological effects of starvation mode, that the overweight or obese experience due to improper fasting.

Changeup Pitch

Obesity's curveball sets the body into experiencing starvation mode, and all the physical feelings of hunger and cravings associated with starvation. These physical symptoms combined with the visual reality of continued weight gain, creates great emotional and psychological stress within us, as we diet or fast improperly. We may be doing everything else right. We may be eating good food and exercising, in essence, we are swinging the bat perfectly, but the timing is off. The cumulative effect of improper fasting or dieting will result in weight gain rather than weight loss. This weight gain sets us over the edge. Eventually, we throw the bat down and decide to quit. Obesity has struck us out!

Obesity's Game Plan vs. the Bases Loaded Game Plan

From the observations of these three pitches, the opposition's game plan becomes evident. Obesity wants us to be in starvation mode 24 hours a day! The Bases Loaded game plan is exactly opposite. The program limits starvation mode to that time when we are asleep.

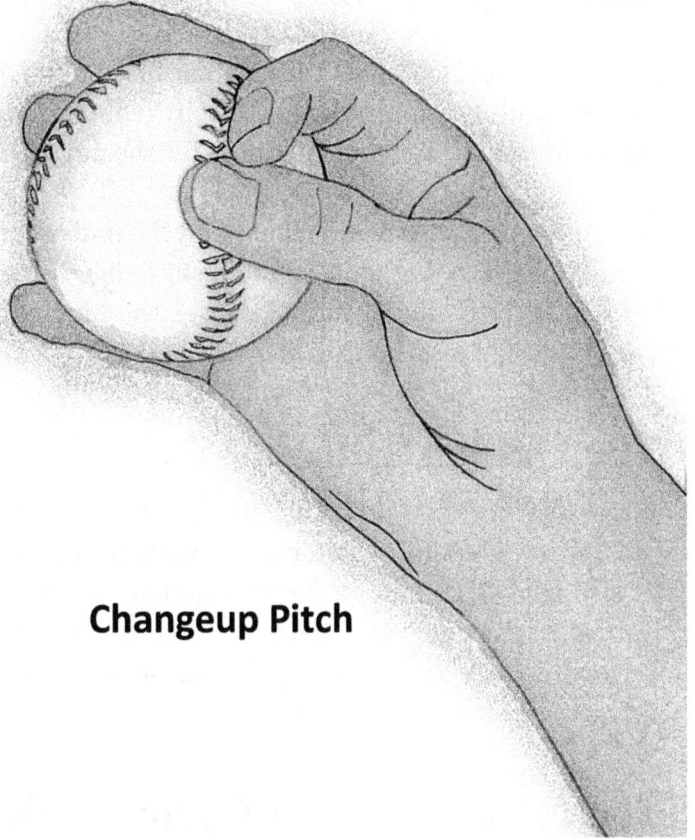

Guarding Against Obesity's Three Pitches

The way to beat Obesity's three pitches is simple; do not strike at the fastball. Breaking the fast in the morning prevents Obesity from throwing his pitches of deception. It enables one to determine metabolism's pace for the day.

By following the Natural Sunset Cycle and doing physical activity in the evening culminating in a workout, metabolism believes its host is making one more search for food. This "positive deception" causes the metabolism to continue burning bright, and leads to weight loss, instead of weight gain.

The Golden Rule and Bases Loaded

Most everyone knows the Golden Rule; "Do unto others as you would have them do unto you." When it comes to interacting with people, it is a good rule to base your life. Let us also apply that rule in the interactions we have with Mr. Metabolism; "Do unto Mr. Metabolism as you would have him do unto you." If we do not let Mr. Metabolism starve during the early part of the day, he will not let us feel starved, and he will also fill us with energy in return as gratitude.

The Natural Sunset Cycle vs. Dieting

The way the body feels during the Natural Sunset Cycle is different from the feelings we feel when we are experiencing "starvation mode" through dieting or improper fasting. During starvation mode, the body of an overweight person is technically not starving. Their body has plenty of reserve fuel on hand. Metabolism, though, makes the mind and body feel that the body is starving. Such a person then feels all the very real feelings that a starving person feels.

During the NS-Cycle, metabolism does not believe the body is starving. As long as we eat the bulk of daily food during the early part of the day, metabolism will not be deceived into believing that the body is in want of fuel. We will feel hungry by the time we go to bed, but we will not feel the lack of energy, irritability and exhaustion throughout the day as a person experiencing starvation mode feels. On the contrary, after a workout and warm shower we will experience a feeling of energy and vitality. Now we might feel exhausted for a split second before sleeping, but soon the alarm bell will awaken us to a delicious short breakfast and a new day!

The Senseless Fight of Dieting

In many ways, the Bases Loaded Plan is a "surrender." It is a giving up and a letting go of one's own will on certain issues, and entrusting one's self to the will of Mr. Metabolism. Mr. Metabolism has been around for quite a while. He knows what he is doing. To fight Mr. Metabolism, to try to put one's will of losing weight over metabolism's will of protecting the body from starvation, amounts to a senseless fight. We might win a battle by losing weight on a crash diet, but the combination of Mr. Metabolism's long-term and short-term memories will eventually work against us. At some point, the combination of a restrictive diet and heavy workouts cause a dieter's metabolism to do something unexpected. The energy demands of a crash diet begin to be interpreted as a threat to the survival of the body. Instead of drawing energy from fat, metabolism starts to draw energy from the body's muscle mass. The body begins the process of protein catabolism.

"People who force themselves to stick with a crash diet will lose bodyweight, but it's a very unfavorable type of weight loss. Typically, half of the pounds lost come from muscle tissue that is sacrificed." [55]

Protein catabolism is a truly puzzling phenomenon that bodybuilders encounter occasionally, but we can explain it with an understanding of metabolism's limited memory. Instead of drawing energy from the reserve fuel tank, an amount of energy that metabolism is unsure about, metabolism chooses to draw energy from muscle tissue. Extracting energy from sacrificed muscle tissue is a slower process than extracting the quick energy available in fat. Thus, protein catabolism can be seen as one of metabolism's energy conservation measures. It slows down energy expenditure and preserves the unknown quantity of quick energy that is available in the reserve storage units. Unfortunately, the process of protein catabolism compromises the dieter's ability to lose weight. Sacrificing muscle also sacrifices the ability of that muscle to burn fat.

"To make matters worse, when you do go off the diet (which everyone who goes on a very low-calorie diet does at some point), you will gain back the fat you lost, and more. That's because you've turned your body into a less efficient fat-burning machine by losing muscle." [56]

Because of limited knowledge concerning metabolism's "limited memory," those who use dieting as a means to lose weight, are putting their body and spirit through a senseless fight. I call it a senseless fight because there is no way to win the war. One can only win battles. There is no such thing as a "victorious dieter." The only slim dieters are those who fight a continuous war with their metabolism. Ironically, such dieters choose to live like the hunter/gatherers by artificially imposing starvation conditions upon themselves. While they may be slim, they are also perpetually hungry like the hunter/gatherers.

Protein Catabolism—The Unseen Enemy

We call protein catabolism the unseen enemy because it is extremely hard for the "overweight" dieter to catch this phenomenon when it occurs. While a thin person will notice the loss of a pound or two of muscle, an overweight person will not notice such a small amount of weight.

In addition to dieting, other stressful factors can combine to cause protein catabolism. These factors include but are not limited to; lack of sleep, lack of adequate nutrition, inadequate protein available to the muscles, sustained heavy exercise, prolonged fasting, prolonged dietary restrictions, or trying to lose weight below ideal weight. Metabolism can interpret any one of these, or a combination of these factors, as a survival threat and induces protein catabolism as an energy conservation measure.

From a theoretical standpoint, protein catabolism is the ultimate folly of modern day dieting. Metabolism is a friend, not an enemy, and yet modern day dieting fights metabolism. How does metabolism react to this fight? Metabolism's only concern is for the survival of its host.

Metabolism has no understanding of the dieter's intentions. Metabolism cannot tell the difference between starvation that occurs when we follow a crash diet, and starvation that occurs when we spend four days searching for food in the wilderness. To metabolism it is all the same, and so the metabolism conserves energy to ensure survival, even if we decide to fight back.

Keep your Eye on the Ball

Attending a baseball practice for beginners, one will hear the coach urging the youngsters to watch the ball, or "Keep your eye on the ball." Often, in the quest to accomplish something worthwhile, we get caught up in the little rules, or we try to take shortcuts. We forget the basics and lose sight of the ball. We lose sight of the big picture. What is the big picture that we want to keep in mind during the Bases Loaded Program? The Bases Loaded Program is the

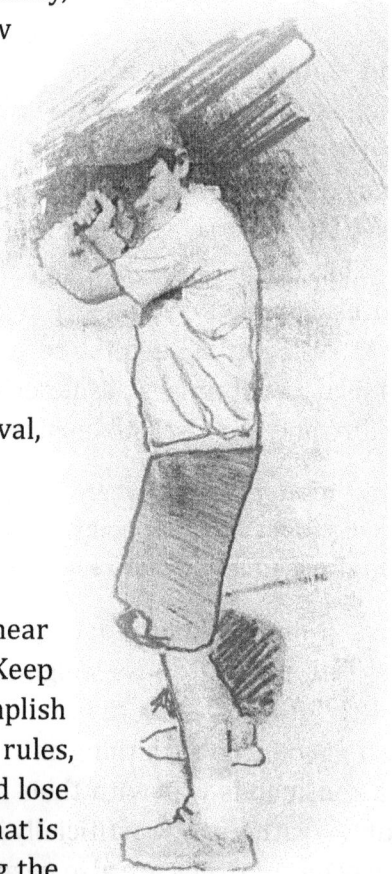

prelude to a whole new way of life. It is a lifestyle change. Remember, we are not trying to outsmart metabolism by resorting to "quick fix" diets that have to be repeated every few months. We are learning to work with the metabolism and not against it. Most importantly, we want children to have a healthy, normal, relationship with food. We want them to learn the principles concerning food that will allow them to take control of their lives. As we have seen from the previous section, not all aspects of hunter/gatherer life are desirable and worthy of emulation. Lack of obesity among the hunter/gatherers was in large part governed by the starvation conditions that they had to endure. Keeping your eye on the ball, and understanding the survival mechanisms programmed into metabolism, enables one to lose weight without resorting to diets that mimic starvation conditions.

Remember, within the Bases Loaded Program, weight loss is imperceptible. Do not be worried about the speed at which weight loss occurs, rather be happy in your direction. Along with the weight loss your forging a special bond with your child. So have fun and be patient with the program. Have a little orange juice, vegetable juice, or prune juice to cut the edge off your hunger at night.

This has been an important chapter. We can see the phenomenon of childhood obesity in a new light. Obesity goes hand in hand with development and modernization of a nation. Obesity happens, in large part because we get caught up in the rush of life and are ignorant of metabolism's rules. American families are trying to run faster than we have the strength to run. Let us slow down the pace. It is probably not a good idea to run the game of life as if it were a "sprint," rather we should run it like a marathon. This chapter has also given us some valuable insights into the deceptive ways of the opponent. We now have a basic plan to beat childhood obesity. Instead of living life continually hungry, we are going to eat from sunrise to sunset and satisfy hunger in a natural way. Instead of thinking about food, we will now be able to focus mental efforts on jobs or schoolwork. We still have some important principles to learn, so review these ideas and come back for some fun!

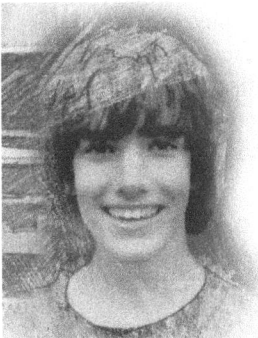

The greatest thing about my program was the fact that I stopped feeling starved throughout the day. Food was available to me from the minute I woke up until early in the evening. I definitely felt better during the day because I was not starving and I think this helped me in my school work. Get good food for your child to eat. Eat during the day instead of late at night. Let them set their own motivation to lose weight. Do not force your kid to lose weight, or punish them if they do not workout. The best thing you can do for your kid in terms of workouts is to have fun with them and actually do the workouts with them.

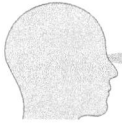

Check Your Understanding

1. **What is Obesity's fastball?**

    Answer: *Obesity's fastball occurs when we fail to observe the Natural Sunset Cycle and fast in the early morning hours.*

2. **What is Obesity's curveball?**

    Answer: *Obesity's curveball refers to the deception that occurs due to metabolism's limited memory. Failing to observe the Natural Sunset Cycle, the mind tells us that we are not starving in the morning, but the metabolism believes otherwise.*

3. **What is Obesity's changeup pitch?**

    Answer: *Obesity's changeup pitch refers to the psychological and emotional stress that occurs as a result of living in a continuous state of starvation mode while continuing to gain weight.*

4. **What is the best thing we can do to guard against Obesity's three pitches?**

    Answer: *Observing the Natural Sunset Cycle will guard against Obesity's three pitches.*

5. **What is the name of the condition where the body breaks down muscle tissue instead of fat, to meet the energy demands of the body?**

    Answer: *Metabolism sometimes uses protein catabolism to conserve energy.*

6. **Explain protein catabolism using an understanding of metabolism's limited memory.**

    Answer: *Improper fasting or unusual stress put upon the human body causes the metabolism to believe the body is starving. Extracting energy from muscle is a slower process than extracting energy from fat. Since metabolism cannot remember the amount of fat reserves, metabolism uses protein catabolism as a conservation measure, to save energy reserves, and slow down the expenditure of energy in an effort to delay starvation.*

7. **How does protein catabolism compound the problem of obesity?**

    Answer: *Since muscle tissue is the means whereby metabolism burns energy, reducing the muscle mass of the body reduces the efficiency of the body to burn fat.*

8. **From the Bases Loaded perspective, why is it important for us to stay away from dieting?**

    Answer: *Dieting has to be a continual process in order to remain slim. Dieters ironically take upon themselves the life of a hunter/gatherer, where they are perpetually hungry and often lack energy through the day. The Bases Loaded Program offers children a new way of life. It allows them to satisfy their hunger and focus their energies away from food. It allows them to develop their talents and become everything that they can be.*

9. **Compare Obesity's game plan to the Bases Loaded game plan.**

    Answer: *Obesity wants us to be in starvation mode 24 hours a day. The Bases Loaded game plan is exactly the opposite. The program limits starvation mode to that time when we are asleep.*

10. **Compare the feeling one has during dieting to the feelings one has observing the Natural Sunset Cycle.**

    Answer: *Observing the Natural Sunset Cycle one will feel hungry by the time they go to sleep, but will not feel the lack of energy, irritability and exhaustion throughout the day that a dieter will feel.*

11. **Why did Joe feel better after the first few weeks of his program?**

    Answer: *Eating a good breakfast and eating the bulk of his food during the day allowed Joe to avoid Obesity's deceptive pitches. He no longer felt starved.*

In terms of physical activity, Bases Loaded is mainly about having physical fun.

A Mountain of Love

Here is a trivia question for you. What is the famous movie that uses baseball as a motif, but is really more about life and the dreams we have in life? Here are a couple paraphrased lines from the movie, clues for you. "Heaven is where your dreams come true." And, from the last scene, "Dad, can we play catch?" Indeed, if we could look into the souls of our children, we might find that their conception of heaven on earth, or "**Field of Dreams**," is as simple as doing something fun with a parent.

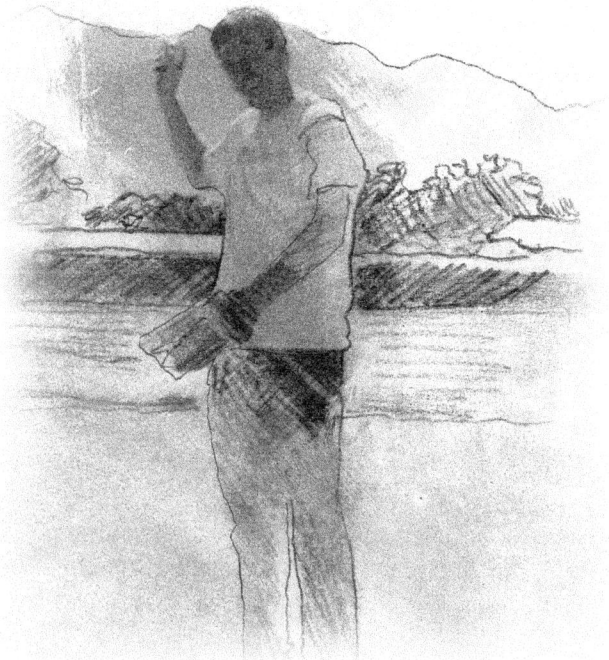

Having Fun

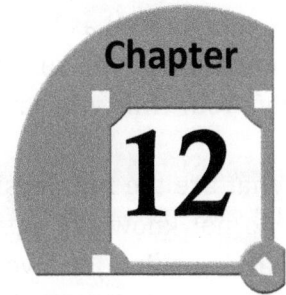

If your family does not have fun the first week doing this program, then please read this chapter once a week until your family starts having fun. Then have fun every week for the rest of your life. Seriously! Most of the adults reading this book have forgotten how to have fun, the fun that one had as a child. You are all grown up and have a grownup attitude. In many ways, your attitude has become like Mr. Metabolism's attitude. Physical activity is no longer fun but just a bunch of work. I converted to a grownup attitude when I was about to start my junior year in high school.

It was a summer football practice. We were running sprints to the point of exhaustion. There were many players throwing up, one even fainted from the heat. It was one of those rare moments of mature teenage introspection, when the thought crossed my mind, "This is not so much fun as it is hard work!" I would not trade my high school football years for anything. The maturity that came from playing high school sports has helped me through life. Sadly, as I grow older, I see coaches teaching this same "work" attitude in sports to younger children. Gone are the sandlot baseball and football games. Children still play these games, but they rarely organize them between themselves. It is all done through the parents. Children cannot even fight on the playing field anymore. That is reserved for the parents, as well. Gone is the fun. It is all about work-work!

Here is an idea to consider. Could it be that there is a correlation between the lack of physical fun in a child's life, and the tendency for that child to become overweight? I think so. Remember what we read about Joe in his short history. He put on the weight in grade 4, when he was stressing at school and lacked confidence. Life was not fun for him. He participated in sports, but even organized sports failed to provide daily physical fun for him. It seems that many children in America are like Joe. In their search for fun, many have chosen to spend endless hours playing video games. Many live their lives in a virtual world devoid of physical activity.

In terms of physical activity, Bases Loaded is mainly about having physical fun. The Bases Loaded Program is about bike rides, throwing the baseball, kicking the soccer ball, or going swimming. It is about running as fast as one can for the sheer joy of running. It can be as complicated as learning a martial art, or as simple as going for a walk or throwing a football. What makes these activities fun for your child? Believe it or not Mom or Dad, it is you. Your child will have fun because they will be doing these activities with their parent.

What are the fun physical activities your child will enjoy? That is a good question, but I do not know the answer. Ask your child this question and let their answer be your starting point. Joe loved baseball when we started his program, so naturally we hit and threw baseballs together. We also went on bike rides and threw the football. He enjoyed swimming, so we went to the local recreation center occasionally. Do whatever your child wants to do, as long as it is physical.

If your child does not want to do anything physical then say; "Let us go on a walk and talk about it." Walking is a great physical activity that keeps metabolism's intensity strong. More importantly, walks are great because of the talking and joking around together two can share.

I remember one cold evening in December Joe, and I went for a walk. It was about three months into his program. We started composing silly poems as we walked and talked together. I still remember one of the poems.

To this day, Joe and I still laugh about this poem. The poem has become a fond memory of a fun experience that we shared together.

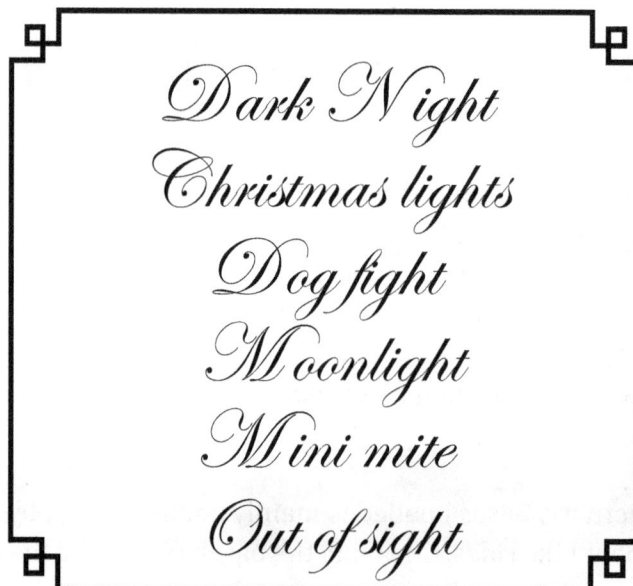

> *Dark Night*
> *Christmas lights*
> *Dog fight*
> *Moonlight*
> *Mini mite*
> *Out of sight*

Become as a Little Child

On one of your morning walks, ponder this question; "Does a child eat to play, or play to eat?" Naturally, a child eats to play. I do not believe parents hear their child say; "Well dad and mom, I would love to go with you right now, but I have a lot of playing to do. How do you expect me to put food on the table if I cannot play?" The above explanation sounds pretty funny. Now substitute the word "play" with the word "work" and it will be clear what I am getting at. Society has taught adults to reverse the natural order of things.

The natural order of things can be seen in the lives of small children. Food is enjoyable and necessary because it allows them to play and have fun in life. As adults, we can learn much from children. We should have the same excitement about life, studies, professions, and roles as parents that children have about play. Food should be enjoyable and bring us pleasure. In the end, though, food is a means whereby we can perform necessary and worthy endeavors. Reversing the natural order of things puts all the emphasis upon food, money and things. Following the natural order, becoming like little children, allows work to become play. We become as the "lilies of the field" which seem not to work and yet are glorious to behold.

The Family Funny Book

Life has many funny moments to balance out the sad. My family has a great way to remember the funny moments. From a good friend, we borrowed the idea of keeping a family funny book. We keep the book in an easy place to find, allowing parents and children the ability to make an entry whenever something funny happens. Consider starting your own family funny book. Your family will not regret it! They say that laughing burns calories. I do not know about that, but I believe humor lightens the spirit. Here are a few entries I found about Joe .

Written by Dad June 1995 (Joe 1 ½ years old) The other day Joe was complaining to the point of tears as if he wanted me to change his diaper again. I had just changed it, so I was confused. I ran upstairs with suspicion in my mind, and sure enough I was right. What I thought was baby ointment, was a tube of mint toothpaste!

Written by Mom July 1999 (Joe 5 years old) Joe unexpectedly was "spotlighted" today during Sunday school. He said his favorite food was pizza. His favorite color was yellow. Then they asked him what he wanted to be when he grew up, and he said "Joe." They asked again, and he said, "Joseph." They asked Dave if he knew what Joe meant and Dave said; "We have been trying to figure that out for 5 years now!"

When to have Fun

When should we have fun? We should have fun right after the last meal of the day. The evenings of big dinners, where family members fill themselves full of food should be rethought. Dinner is a particularly important part of the day for American families. In many cases, it is the only time of the day when all members of the family come together and share their experiences of the day. In the BL- Plan, we want to emphasize the social aspect of dinner, and diminish the tendency for this time to be a pit-stop for refueling the body. Dinner should be modest in size so that physical activity is acceptable and even enjoyable right after we eat. If we have to sleep on the couch after dinner, then we are forfeiting the most important time that we have with children. After dinner, the metabolism will want to slow down. By doing something physical, we will keep the metabolism strong.

"As physiologist Melanie Roffers, PhD, puts it, ""Exercising at this time of the day elevates the metabolic rate just as it's winding down."" Light evening activity also may alleviate late-night cravings for high fat foods."[57]

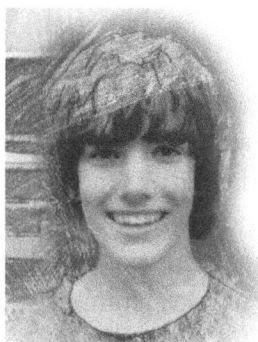

I remember some fun things from my program. I enjoyed biking and running around the yard with our dog Suzy. I liked playing baseball, hockey and passing the football. We probably played more baseball than all the other things put together. Some activities, like biking, wore me out. As I began to lose weight, the activities didn't seem like part of my program. Fun activities are the best way to get your kid to willingly exercise. Baseball, soccer, hockey (now my personal favorite), football, bike riding, and swimming are some of the things my dad, and I did together. Sometimes my brothers would play with us. Have your kid do things that are fun. Do the activities whenever you can, especially after dinner. This activity counts as a workout if you build up a sweat!

Separate Yourselves from Food

Physical activity right after dinner also presents a great opportunity to signal the beginning of the Natural Sunset Cycle. Finishing dinner and clearing the table separates the family from food. If your family eats dessert after dinner, here is a suggestion. Do dessert the Chinese way. The Chinese people love to finish their meals with cut up oranges. Citrus fruit is very refreshing and will cut any lingering hunger a person might have. So, clear the table of dinner plates and cut up some oranges! Let these oranges be the dessert, or last snack of the day. They can be eaten before or after the fun activity. How long should the fun last? That will depend on a few things. If it is a school evening, perhaps there is homework and the physical activity will last a half hour. If it is summer break or a weekend, perhaps the activity will last over an hour. Since the activity will be fun, we will want to keep playing. We just need to be home before dark, so the rest of the family does not worry.

Keeping Metabolism Strong

When a child has a healthy breakfast, lunch, and participates in normal physical activities at school, their metabolism will burn strong and bright during the day. Activities like walking to class, recess, games in PE class, are low and moderate physical activities that convince metabolism that the body is looking for food. Since Mr. Metabolism ate breakfast, he will gladly expend more energy knowing there is plenty to spare and more is on the way.

Remember, metabolism has no memory of its reserve fuel, only what it has been given that day. Thus, it is this combination of recently consumed food and physical activity that allows metabolism to work and burn energy at a high capacity. In the afternoon, your child is still awake, not yawning in class, and not famished from lack of food, but by dinner, your child's metabolism is starting to taper down. At this point in time, a large meal will not make metabolism grow in intensity as it did earlier in the day. Metabolism's clock is signaling the body to prepare for sleep. The only option we have, to keep metabolism burning bright, is physical activity. By engaging the body in physical activity at this hour of the day, we prevent metabolism from tapering down to conservation mode. Make this physical activity fun for your child and your child will gladly participate in the activity. They will actually look forward to this very critical time of the day.

Keeping Energy Levels Strong

Let us revisit an earlier visual and look at it in terms of keeping metabolism strong through the evening. In the next visual **(Figure 34)**, the dark shade represents food. The medium shade represents metabolism, but also represents the energy level one feels throughout the day. Notice the difference when we compare it to Joe's old lifestyle. The combination of eating early in the morning, and mixing in some low and moderate physical activities throughout the day keeps metabolism's intensity level high.

In the early evening, metabolism desires to slow down. Large amounts of food at this hour of the afternoon will not prevent metabolism from slowing down. We will keep metabolism strong by having a small dinner followed by fun physical activities. Shifting the main meal to an earlier time and having a smaller meal for dinner, is a good plan that offers other health benefits, as well.

"According to researchers, one reason the French have a much lower incidence of heart disease than Americans is that the French have their main meal earlier in the day and then follow it with physical activity."[58]

Finish the evening by doing a short workout to keep the metabolism energy level strong until it is time to go to sleep.

Comparing Energy Levels

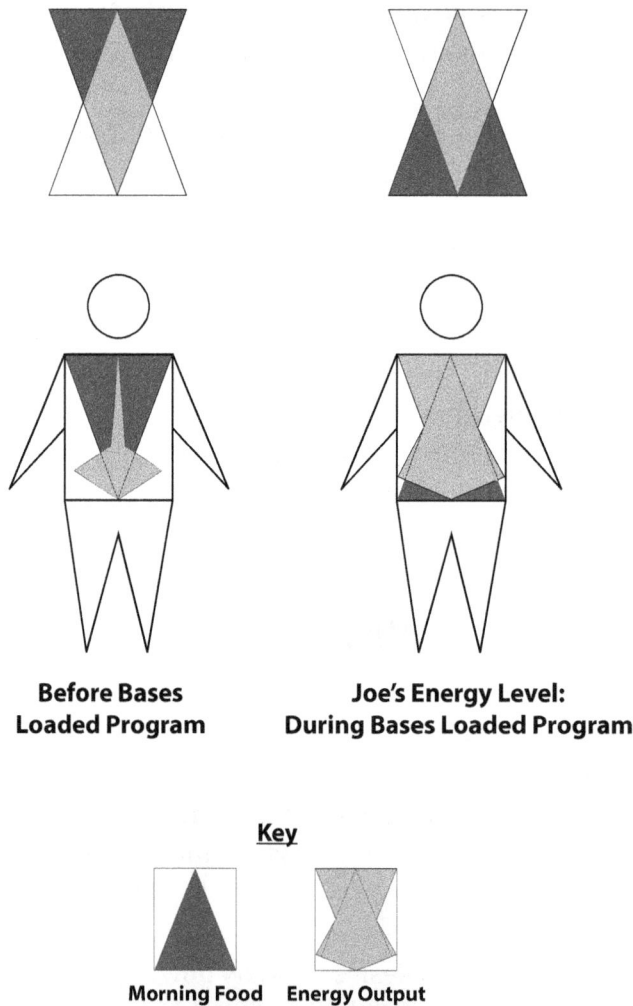

| Before Bases Loaded Program | Joe's Energy Level: During Bases Loaded Program |

Key

Morning Food   Energy Output

Figure 34: Comparing Energy Levels - The medium shade not only represents metabolism, it also represents energy levels. Comparing the two, we find that Joe's energy level was much higher while following the BL-Plan.

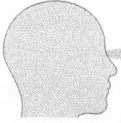

Check Your Understanding

1. **In terms of physical activity, what is the main philosophy of the Bases Loaded Program?**

    Answer: *Parent and child should engage in physical fun together.*

2. **What are the physical activities that a parent and child should do together?**

    Answer: *Doing the physical activities that are fun for the child should be the priority.*

3. **If a child cannot decide about a physical activity, what activity acts as the default?**

    Answer: *Walking is a great physical activity that allows parent and child to bond.*

4. **When should fun physical activities take place?**

    Answer: *Fun physical activities should be done right after dinner.*

5. **How long should physical activities last?**

    Answer: *Physical activities should last 1/2 to 3 hours depending on schedule.*

6. **Why is it so important to do these activities after dinner?**

    Answer: *Metabolism is starting to slow down at this time and physical activity will prolong metabolism's intensity.*

7. **Will food consumption in the evening stimulate metabolism to burn more energy?**

    Answer: *Without physical activity, food consumed in the evening converts to fat.*

8. **Should large meals occur in the evening?**

    Answer: *No, large meals need to occur earlier in the day, meals at dinner should be much smaller.*

9. **How does lack of physical fun contribute to obesity?**

    Answer: *Lack of physical fun inhibits stress release and causes children to turn to more passive forms of entertainment like video games.*

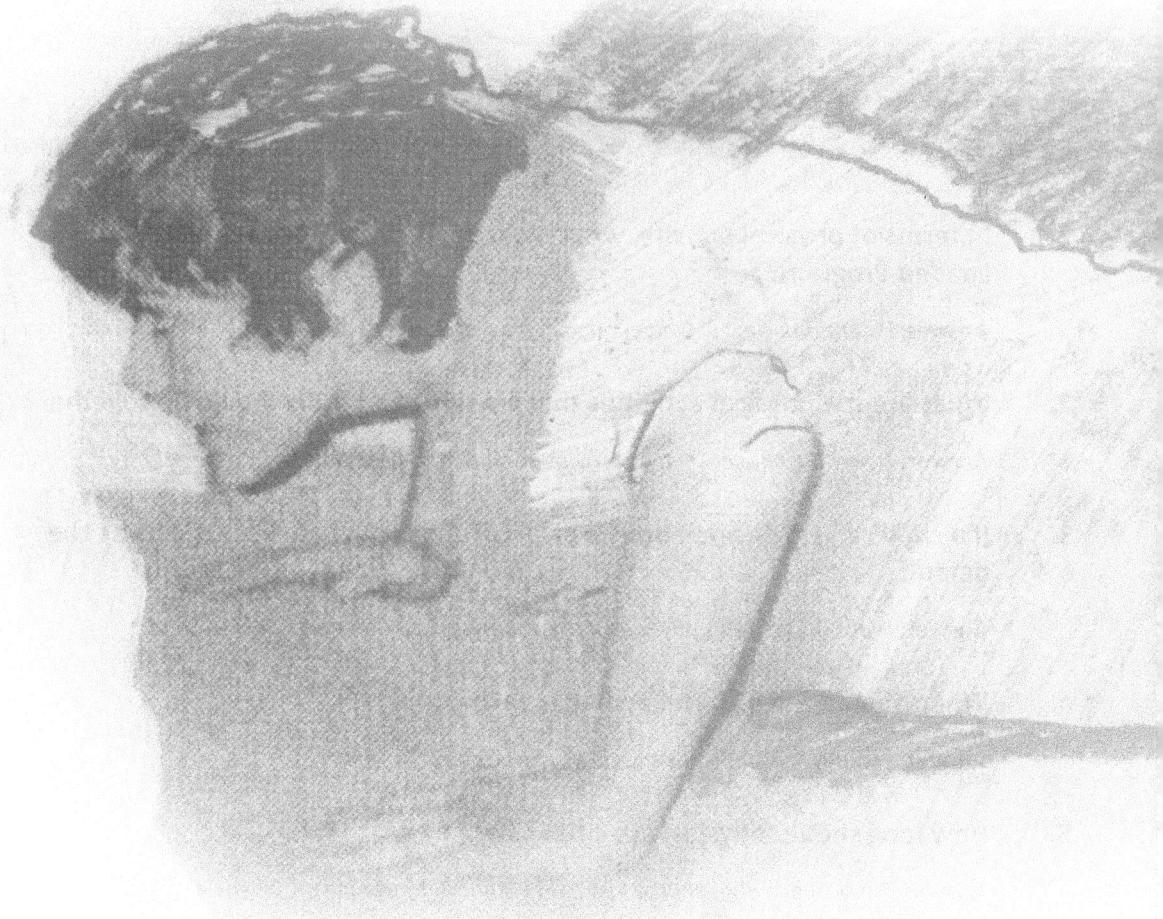

Exercise combinations are a lot like food combinations. Getting a variety of exercise helps to nourish the muscles of the body.

Work-ins and Workouts

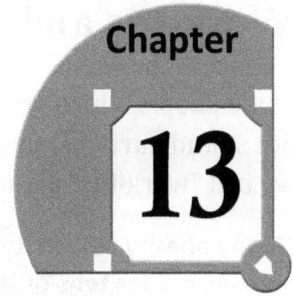

Let us define some terms. By the term "work-ins" we are referring to conscious and unconscious movements of the body that cause the metabolism to build in intensity but do not expend a lot of energy in the process. A "workout" is a physical activity that causes the metabolism to grow in intensity to full capacity. A workout will cause the metabolism to expend a great amount of energy. It is a predetermined set of exercises or physical activity that will put stress on the muscles of the body. A good way to remember the difference is to think about sweat. Workouts make the sweat come "out" of the body while work-ins keep the sweat "in" the body. Within the course of a day, we will try to push the body to accomplish one workout. We will try to time this workout so that it occurs at the end of the waking hours, right before we go to sleep.

Work-ins

The BL-Program advocates doing as many daily work-ins as possible. I have never counted the amount of work-ins that Joe or I have accomplished in the course of a day. I imagine that the number exceeds several hundred. Some work-ins include, walking up the stairs, taking out the garbage, mowing the lawn, setting the table, getting the mail or anything else that requires physical movement by the body. Along with these unconscious work-ins, we add conscious activities such as stretching, going for a walk after breakfast, doing 15 push-ups during a commercial break, or 15 sit-ups before having a snack. We can also add fun activities to the list such as riding a bike, throwing a football, or having a water balloon fight. Not only are there no restrictions in terms of quantity, but there are no time restrictions associated with work-ins. We can work the body in this manner anytime day or night. Since we are not working the body extremely hard, we can do these activities right after we eat. Be creative! Work in the garden. Clean the house, or work on the things contained in the perennial "things to do" list. Doing the "to do" list, men, will certainly please your wife and perhaps lead to certain physical activities that a couple can enjoy together!

Work-Ins and the Hunter/Gatherers

Some people who love to workout are probably saying, "This whole work-in concept does not sound particularly significant!" On the contrary, the latest research shows that what we call "work-ins" actually permeated the lives of the hunter/gatherers.

"Many obesity researchers now believe that very frequent low level physical activity—the kind humans did for tens of thousands of years before the leaf blower was invented—may actually work better for us than the occasional bouts of exercise you get as a gym rat." [59]

Why is this low level physical activity required in the fight against obesity? We discussed this issue in the last chapter as it relates to the metabolism model. Now let us look at the issue in greater detail as it relates to the fact that human beings are biologically and genetically patterned after the hunter/gatherers. Let us consider the lives of the hunter/gatherers.

Did the hunter/gathers spend all of their time running at full speed in pursuit of their prey? No, they spent most of their time preparing for the hunt. They had to walk around the wilderness, to find materials to make weapons or traps. They made those weapons and traps using their arm and hand muscles. They had to walk and search for their prey. When they found it, they had to walk as quietly as possible to get within range of throwing a spear, boomerang, or shooting an arrow. Once they killed their prey, they then had to carry or drag it. When they returned to camp, they had to prepare their catch into a meal. They had to gut the animal, skin it, create a fire, and cook the meat. While the men were out hunting, the women were probably busy gathering. Gathering required walking, searching, picking, bending of the back, get-on-your-hands-and-knees type of work.

After gathering, everything had to be carried back to base camp. They then prepared the gathered items for eating. After the eating of the meal when darkness set in, the hunter/gatherers did not go directly to sleep. No, indeed, art lessons had to be taught to the children. Everyone retired to the cave with fire sticks. They prepared dyes and created beautiful cave paintings depicting the day's hunt. I am sure there are many more things that I am leaving out here, but I think one can see what I am trying to say. If we were to take away all of the low and moderate level physical activities involved in the above scenario, we would be left with only a few physically stressful activities. The activities associated with killing an animal, such as running and throwing a weapon would constitute a workout. Dragging an animal carcass for a portion of the journey home would be even more physically demanding.

Still, one can see, that most of the physical activities of the hunter/gatherers were low to moderate by modern day standards. The important concept to grasp here is the fact that these physical activities took up most of the day. The hunter/gatherers were constantly moving. Their survival depended on this physical movement.

We of the present age are like the hunter/gatherers. The modern day metabolism responds very well to low and moderate level physical activity or movement. Metabolism believes these expenditures of energy are essential for survival. Thus, food consumed early in the day, intermingled with work-ins sends the signal to metabolism, to burn lots and lots of fuel. Metabolism "invests" this high expenditure of fuel for a greater return.

Work-Ins and America

As we discussed earlier, Mr. Metabolism is blind when it comes to food and physical activity. He believes that when we are playing catch or raking leaves that we are preparing for a hunt. Let us follow this line of analysis a little longer. I think that we will begin to see just how powerful work-ins are in the fight against obesity. Let us do a very quick historical profile of American work-ins.

Farmers and ranchers settled America. Think of the activities of those who worked the farms and ranches. In those days, working the fields and taking care of the animals required physical movement. This physical movement was hard work. It was a combination of work-ins and workouts that began in the morning and ended when the sun went down. The main meal of the day was in the afternoon. The combination of daytime food and constant physical movement made metabolism strong. This strength was reflected in their physical bodies. Obesity was nonexistent among these types of workers. As America became a modern nation, the population shifted towards the cities. Workers manned the factories, craftsmen and builders set up businesses. Men continued to work "from sun to sun" while the work of the women "was never done." Physical activity still dominated the lives of the average American. Food was for the most part wholesome and unprocessed during the first half of the 20th century. Again we see the same three-way relationship working for the good of Americans. Food was wholesome. Americans ate and physically moved around during the day. This physical movement consisted of work-ins mixed with occasional workouts that took up most of the day. Obesity was minimal.

America prospered and leisure time increased. How did Americans fill their leisure time? Believe it or not the great American pastime was not football, rather baseball. Historically, baseball has pastoral roots, offering its earliest participants leisurely diversion from the hard work of the fields. Players run the bases, or chase a ball, but mostly baseball is a game of skill and physical fun.

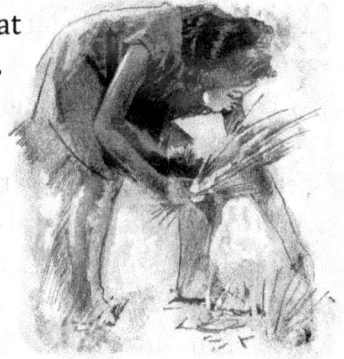

In many respects, baseball is much like the hunt and the preparation of the hunt that the hunter/gatherers experienced. In baseball, the players even get to carry around a club shaped like the earliest of hunter/gatherer weapons!

The second half of the 20th century, after WWII, saw many changes to American society. We have already spoken of the changes that occurred in food. As food became less nutritious and more refined, the killers, cancer and heart disease, increased. From 1945 to 1980, factory workers steadily declined. In terms of work-ins, this meant that daily physical movement decreased in the workplace. The incidence of obesity slowly increased with all these changes.

During the second half of the century, Americans compensated for the lack of physical movement during the day with more rigorous physical activities during their free time. In other words, as work-ins decreased, workouts took their place. It was as if we were taking all the work-ins that the body ached for during the day, and squeezed them into an available 30-minute workout slot. During the early part of this time, (my growing-up years) the great American pastime of baseball diminished in popularity. Sports requiring more rigorous physical conditioning such as football, soccer and hockey, increased in popularity. Individual sports took on greater importance. Weight lifting, jogging and long distance running became very popular in the 70's.

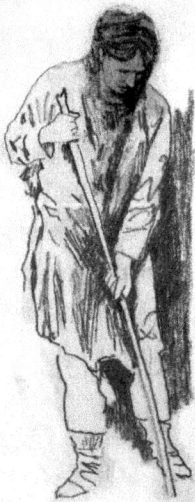

With the advent of the computer age, from the late 1980's to present, this trend to gravitate away from work-ins towards workouts has accelerated.

"We all need to move more-the Centers for Disease Control and Prevention says our leisure-time physical activity (including things like golfing, gardening, and walking) has decreased since the late 1980's, right around the time the gym boom really exploded."[60]

While Americans are becoming more "workout" oriented, research shows they are also becoming more obese.

"Still, as one major study—the Minnesota Heart Survey—found, more of us at least say we exercise regularly. The survey ran from 1980, when only 47% of respondents said they engaged in regular exercise, to 2000, when the figure had grown to 57%. And yet obesity figures have risen dramatically in the same period: a third of Americans are obese, and another third count as overweight by the Federal Government's definition." [61]

There is a definite correlation then, between the loss of the low and moderate physical activities , the increase of workouts, and the incidence of obesity.

Does this mean we should stop doing workouts and do work-ins? I do not think so. We cannot put the blame on workouts. As discussed earlier, that in terms of obesity among children, the computer age, with its virtual games and entertainment, has done its part to take children away from the fun "physical" games, or work-ins, that characterized the leisure time of generations past. When one thinks about it from the perspective of Mr. Metabolism, the puzzle pieces come together. Mr. Metabolism was programmed for both the hunt and the preparation of the hunt. Both work-ins and workouts are vital. If one of these is missing or we try to replace one with the other, it has an effect on metabolism.

A good way to think of it is to picture in your mind a huge campfire. The burning bright flames represent metabolism. Think about the making of that huge fire. It started with little shavings of wood and a small flame. They added small pieces of wood (kindling) and finally the big logs. In this example, we can compare the small shavings and small pieces of wood to work-ins. The big logs can be compared to a workout. Can we make a large fire with only the big logs? No, but that is exactly what we are trying to do when we replace work-ins with a workout. Can we build a fire with the shavings and kindling only? Yes, we can, but it will not be as large of a fire without some big logs included. With the image of the huge campfire in mind, the value of both work-ins and workouts becomes apparent. We are now in a position to take a closer look at the big logs, or workouts.

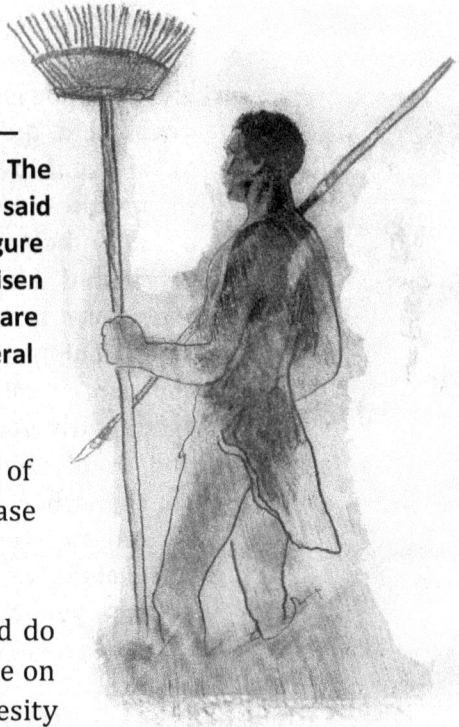

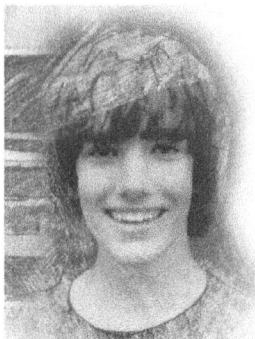

Because I was home-schooled during my program, I was able to combine my exercises and my snacking together. I got into the habit of doing an exercise before grabbing a snack. I did an exercise (push-ups, sit-ups, bicycles) every 30 minutes, grabbed a quick snack, and then went back to my studies. I never went overboard on these little exercises. I never tried to break a sweat. I think that these little mini workouts actually helped me study better. My dad and I talked about ways that kids at school can do more exercises. We decided that they probably get plenty of exercise by walking in the halls, doing PE, or if they are smaller—having recess. But you can do more; maybe you can explain the program you are doing with your teachers. Stay after class for just a minute and do a quick exercise like push-ups or jumping jacks when all the other kids have cleared the class. Hurry to your next period by walking very fast. If any of your friends catch you doing the push-ups, just tell them that your teacher is helping you to lose weight.

Work-ins and Workouts with Suzy the Dog

I am not an animal scientist, but it seems that dogs, and probably most warm-blooded animals, share the same type of metabolism as humans. I base my opinion on observations I made of my family's pet dog Suzy. These observations show the close relationship that work-ins and workouts share. Suzy is about five years old. When we got her, she was a truly active puppy. Her favorite activities included digging holes in the lawn as well as chewing up everything in sight. When we took her for a walk it was more like her taking us for a run. She would strain and pull us along by the leash. About a year ago she slowed down. She gained weight and seemed bored with life. She still enjoyed walks, but walked with us instead of pulling us along. After her walks, she would sit down in the shade where she would lie for hours.

We decided to buy a new puppy for the little children and thought that Suzy might enjoy a playmate, as well. We were right! Suzy followed that little puppy around everywhere. It was comical to see the two dogs playing with each other. Suzy was twice the size of Tink, the new dog. They played in the back yard looking like heavyweight and flyweight wrestlers going after each other. This playing went on all day. Within a few weeks, it was apparent that Suzy had lost a lot of weight. She had a faster pace in her walks and seemed to be happier about life.

As my wife and I pondered the reason why Suzy had lost so much weight, we could only note two real changes in Suzy's routine since we bought Tink. First, Suzy was eating more food. We caught her eating Tink's food when her food ran out. How could eating more food make her lose weight? She still enjoyed two walks (workouts) a day that made her sweat and made her get out of breath, that had not changed. The only other real change was the constant play (work-ins) she enjoyed. Workouts alone were not enough to keep the weight off of Suzy. When the small constant seemingly insignificant movements, or work-ins, replaced the inactivity of lying in the shade, that is when Suzy lost the weight.

Work-ins and Parents

Those that sit all day at a job will probably feel pretty tired by the end of the workday. Tiredness has to do with the metabolism. Metabolism interprets inactivity and low light, the kind of indoor light enjoyed at work, as signals of hibernation. Under these conditions, metabolism believes that its host is curling up in a cave for a winter's nap. Since metabolism does not know how long it will be before awaking from the winter's nap, the lack of energy indicates metabolism's job of conserving energy.

Incorporating conscious work-ins during the workday, will not only help one lose weight, but will also help one be a better employee. Increasing metabolism intensity brings energy to both mind and body. Here is an idea. Bring a little alarm clock to work. Set the alarm clock to go off at the beginning of every hour. When the alarm goes off, take a few moments and climb a flight of stairs or walk around. If your workplace is a small area, do some isometric exercises and stretches. Do work-ins, and things will work out!

Workouts

Now we have come to the most important part for all of those who love to sweat! Yes, we will speak about workouts. Believe it or not, I love to sweat, so I am speaking from experience. There is something addicting about a good workout. Workouts push the body to the point of stress, where one has to breathe faster. Workouts cause one to sweat from the heat the body generates. The reason that workouts become addicting has to do with the good feelings we have after a workout. The body produces hormones during a workout that gives one a sense

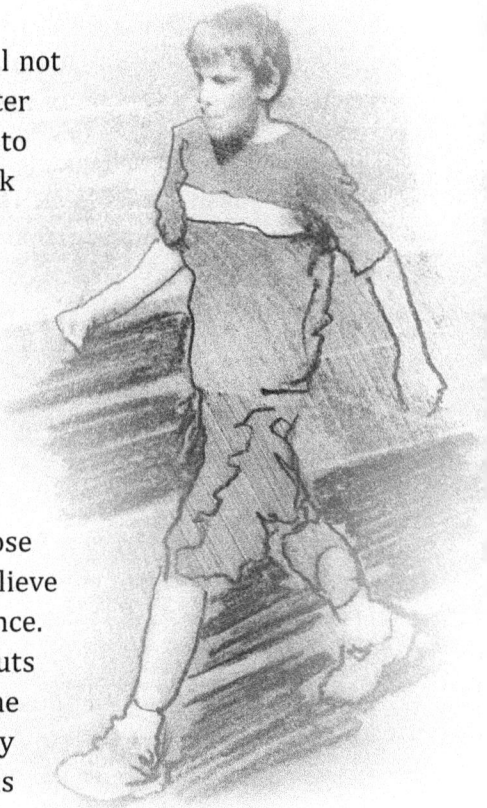

of newness. The word "recreation," derives from this feeling of newness after a workout. We in a sense re-create ourselves from strenuous physical activity.

Why would the body reward us with good feelings after a workout? The answer is simple. Metabolism is programmed for survival, and so is the physical body. The physical body rewards itself for doing those things, which ensure its own survival. A good workout and the rest after that workout make the body stronger. The body can move faster, jump higher, and run away from angry animals that would like to hurt us while we are out hunting and gathering food.

Ever hunt with a bow and arrow on horseback or gather your buddies and hunt buffalo on foot with nothing more than spears made from sharpened rock? I have not been privileged to do either of the above. I can imagine that both experiences would require an incredible amount of physical endurance, flexibility, and strength. Modern day workouts then mimic the workouts that hunter/gatherers received during the hunt.

There is another reward that comes from doing a daily workout. Mr. Metabolism actually gets stronger. Research has proven that the resting metabolic rate correlates to the lean body weight, or muscle of the body.

"By strengthening and toning your muscles, you raise your resting metabolic rate, the one that keeps your body running smoothly even when you are sedentary." [62]

In other words, workouts help the body develop muscle, which in turn increase metabolism's idle speed (resting metabolic rate). Herein we answer a question posed in the beginning of this book. Why is it that some people have a higher idle speed for their metabolism than others? Toning and strengthening the muscles of the body through exercise is the answer. Some may be confused right now thinking, "I thought hard physical work caused metabolism to slow down, not speed up!" Clarification needs to be made here. Recall from the visual studies that we looked at earlier that metabolism slowed down after a hard

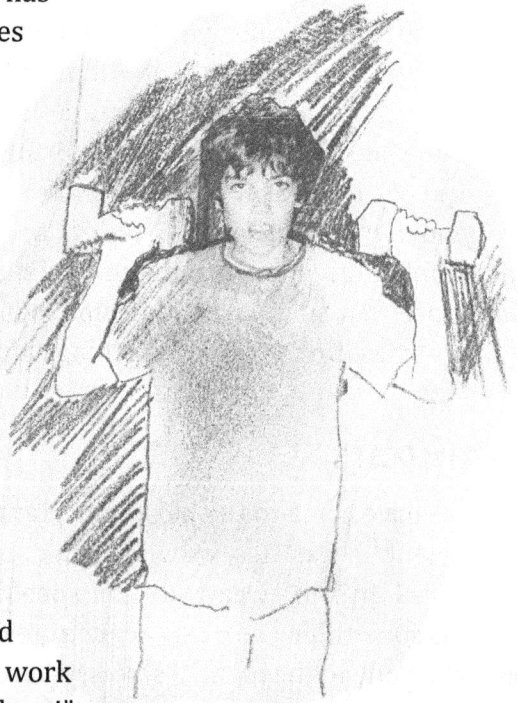

physical workout. Remember that this slowdown occurred because the body went through this workout without having any food in the early part of the day. Metabolism slows down for two reasons. It slows down when the body is preparing for sleep, and it also slows down if it believes the body is starving. It is the combination of hard physical work and lack of food that mimics the conditions of starvation and reduces metabolism to conservation speed.

In terms of the physical activity portion of the program, the daily workout becomes a very significant feature. With every other element of the program in place, the daily workout will convince metabolism that we truly are doing that which the body has been programmed to do. We are hunter/gatherers, worthy of metabolism's full cooperation.

When to do Workouts

Workouts should be done at the end of the evening, when the body has digested its daily food. For those parents that do a workout in the morning, it may be hard to imagine doing a workout at the end of the evening. Be assured that, eating a modest sized dinner and following that dinner with a fun physical activity or other types of work-ins, the metabolism will provide plenty of energy to begin and sustain a workout. Evening workouts have another advantage over the morning or afternoon workout. Remember, Mr. Metabolism has a whole different attitude at the end of the evening than he has during the morning and early afternoon hours. In the early part of the day, metabolism wants food. At the end of the evening metabolism wants to go to sleep. Knowing this, what kind of feelings will a person feel after a morning workout? Mr. Metabolism is going to make that person feel extra hungry.

"The basic problem is that while it's true that exercise burns calories and that you must burn calories to lose weight, exercise has another effect: it can stimulate hunger. That causes us to eat more, which in turn can negate the weight-loss benefits we just accrued." [63]

While it is true that sometimes we may feel hungry at the end of the night, after a workout, it is nothing like the hunger one feels after a workout during the day. Remember, metabolism believes that your heavy workout in the daytime was the result of a hunt and a catch. The strong feeling of hunger we feel after a daylight workout is Mr. Metabolism's method of making sure we eat the catch that he so graciously provided the energy to obtain. What is the feeling the metabolism gives us after a late night workout? The dominant feeling that we will hold after an evening workout is a sense of exhaustion! It is a good sense of exhaustion. It is a feeling of satisfaction that we gave the day 100% effort, both physically and mentally.

Mr. Metabolism's concern is not with food at the end of the evening. He mainly just wants to go to sleep! Here is a good question; "Are we not behaving more like hunter/gatherers by doing our workouts in the daytime and eating a large meal afterwards?" My answer to that question would be; "Yes, and that is precisely the reason that those who do daytime workouts are at a disadvantage in the realm of weight loss!"

By performing a workout, and following that workout with a big meal, one is following their instincts. One is doing, exactly that, which the hunter/gatherers did. There is one difference. While the hunter/gatherers were lucky to get a good catch occasionally, we are able to perform the ritual of the hunt and feast daily. No doubt the hunter/gatherers hunted their prey during the day and ate their feast as soon as possible. Sometimes this feast was during the day but most often it was during the evening hours. No matter the time, they gained several pounds after their feast. They were pounds that kept them alive several days or even weeks when meat was scarce, and they had to rely on gathered items, to keep them alive until the next successful hunt.

Why is it that Americans are working out more, but obesity statistics continue to go up? As we learned earlier, Americans have forsaken an important instinctual urge (work-ins). We can now add to that another reason. Americans are a little too zealous at following other instinctual urges (eating patterns of the hunter/gatherers). Ironically, morning, afternoon and early evening workouts have worked to America's disadvantage. Lacking understanding of metabolism's clock, these workouts have pushed "eating times" into the evening hours when metabolism wants to go to sleep. Put in other words, the food that we eat right after an early morning workout is not so much the problem, but it is the fact that we delay eating time, and we tend to eat in 12-hour cycles that creates the problem. If a person does not eat until 11:00 a.m., then they tend to eat until 11:00 p.m. If one engages in an afternoon or early evening workout, that person will most likely follow their instinctual urge and eat a large dinner right when metabolism slows down for the evening. Granted, the nightly workout is one aspect of the Bases Loaded Program that is not in keeping with the lifestyle of the ancient hunter/gatherers. Keep in mind that it is a temporary condition. Once we achieve the goal of ideal weight, we will reduce late evening workouts.

After the BL-Program, we will maintain ideal weight through an active lifestyle as well as following the natural cycles regarding food. The family lifestyle will be similar to that of your great-great grandparents generation in certain ways.

The late night workout offers many advantages. Let us recount them. When we awake in the morning, there is no need to delay food. By eating early, we will be following the 12-hour eating cycle that the body naturally prefers. We will eat from sun to sun instead of noon to midnight. We will have more energy during the day because we are building the metabolism fire with small shavings and kindling (work-ins), rather than big logs (workout). At night, after the workout, exhaustion comes right before going to sleep rather than right after dinner. Best of all we can fall asleep being a gram or two lighter, rather than the same weight that we have maintained for several years under the daylight workout plan.

Workout What and How

End of the night workouts should not be long; twenty to twenty-five minutes is all we need. Any type of physical activity is acceptable, as long as the workout causes us to breathe harder and build up a sweat. Before the workout begins, stretch the muscles of the body, especially those muscles that you are going to use in your workout. A workout should start out slow and build in intensity. The last minute of a particular exercise or workout should be the most intense. If one chooses to walk fast for a workout, then that person should try to jog for the last minute.

If one jogs for a workout, then that person should try to sprint for the last minute. If doing a series of exercises for twenty minutes, like push-ups, sit-ups, deep knee bends, pull-ups, leg lifts, then limit each exercise to one set. Do as many of each exercise as possible.

For example, start your exercise routine with push-ups. The first few push-ups will warm up the muscles. We keep doing push-ups until we cannot do any more. We stop at this point, when the arms are extended straight and take 4 deep breaths. The body will seem to have a little more energy than before the deep breaths. Push yourself to do 5 or 10 more. These last few push-ups will work muscles intensely. After finishing pushups, rest for a minute and then move on to the next exercise like sit-ups. Follow the pattern described above for each exercise. Twenty minutes of this kind of physical activity will give the body a very good workout. Following the workout, stretch the muscles once again as the body cools down.

Vary the workouts, and try not to do the same thing two nights in a row. If one lifts weights on Monday, that person can do aerobics on Tuesday. Maybe lift weights again on Wednesday, but this time work on the leg muscles instead of the upper body. Exercise combinations are a lot like food combinations.

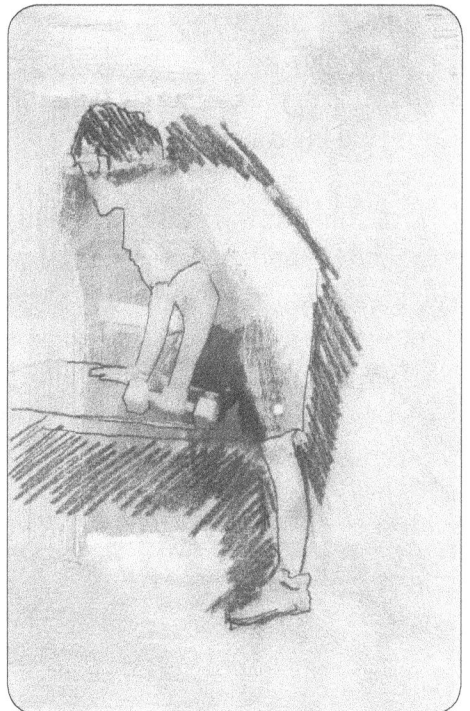

Getting a variety of exercise helps to nourish the muscles of the body.

Encourage your child towards improvement, but do it in a game situation. "I bet you cannot do 5 push-ups!" "I can too!" "Okay, then prove it to me! Wow, you proved me wrong!"

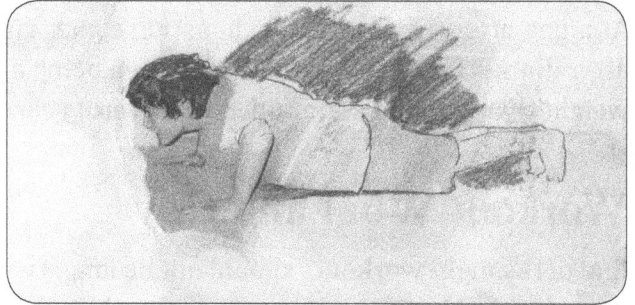

Believe it or not, it is part of human nature to improve oneself. Why? I believe that we are programmed that way to ensure survival. As I mentioned earlier, from Mr. Metabolism's perspective, we all have the need to become better physically to ensure the body's survival.

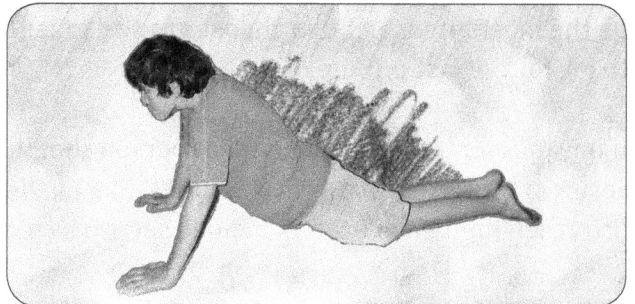

Improvement happens at a slow pace. For example, Joe could only do one full push-up at the beginning of his program. We, therefore, switched him to modified push-ups where he kept his knees on the ground. As time passed, and he lost weight, he was able to switch back to regular push-ups. After a years time, he was able to do 12 full push-ups. Imagine how this improvement boosted his confidence.

Have fun! I know that some believe that we should not have fun during workouts. I, on the other hand, believe that the words of my Aunt Mary apply here, "A spoonful of sugar makes the medicine go down." Children must have an odd sense of humor because they think that it is fun to do things with their parents. This especially applies to physical activities and even workouts. Perhaps children enjoy seeing their parents sweat. So, turn up the volume on the TV and sweat to your favorite workout videos. Remember, work becomes play when we do work together.

More from the Funny Book

Nov. 2000 (Joe 6 years old) I have been telling Joe that he is the apple of my eye. He thinks that is funny. The other day he came up to me and said, "Mom, you are the green apple in my eye!"

Jan. 2000 (Joe 6 years old) A few days ago Joe took a flying saucer toy that had a bubble thing in the middle of it. He then asked me to cut pieces of black and red paper, then he wrote numbers on the papers, and taped the numbers around the middle of the toy. Then he started the toy turning on the kitchen floor and threw a white marble in it. He waited till the toy stopped revolving and he called out the number that the marble landed. Joe had made a roulette wheel! He had seen one in a cartoon and decided all by himself to make it!

Workouts with Coach Tuff AzNails

Understanding that metabolism intensity is contingent upon the two variables of food and physical activity, empowers a person to make wise decisions concerning workouts. For example, let us say your children love to play hockey. They enjoy playing it so much that they want to join an organized team. This is great! They are now enrolled in a fun activity that involves hard physical work. What should a parent do in the following situations?

One child's coach, coach Tuff AzNails, wants the team to have a hard physical hockey practice early Saturday morning. No use trying to convince Coach to change his training time to late evening. The "ice" time cannot be changed. No use trying to get food in your child before practice. The hard physical workout would cause them to throw-up all over the ice. Get some food in your child after the practice, as soon as they are hungry. Their metabolism will interpret this workout as a successful quest for food and will continue to burn brightly.

What if the practice starts at 6:00 p.m., during dinner? Get some food in your child 2-3 hours prior to practice. Give your child an early dinner, and then feed your child a large snack or a small meal after practice.

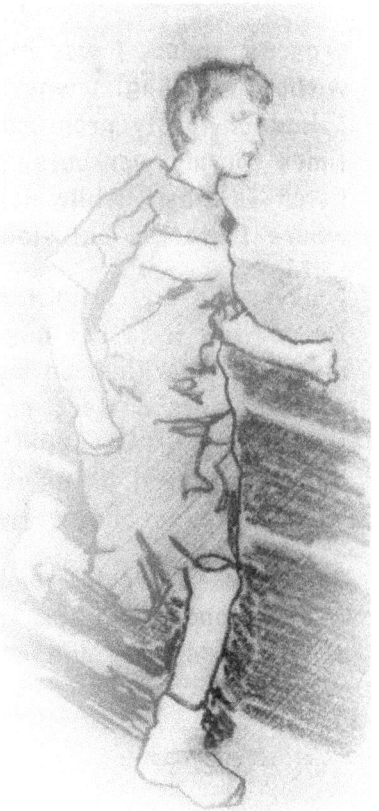

Whenever your child has a hard physical workout during the day, do not require them to have another workout at the end of the evening. Realize that the workout your child has in a game or scrimmage is comparable to the workout of a buffalo hunt. This type of workout will be far more intense than a preconceived workout because your child will be doing fun things. Respect the buffalo hunt that your child has accomplished. At the end of the evening, instead of a workout, do a work-in together. Go on a walk around the track at the fitness center. Talk about the events of the buffalo hunt and point out all the good things your child did during the event.

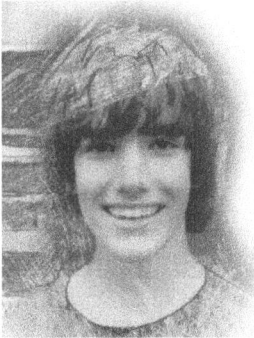

When I first started my program, it seemed like everything that I did was a workout. Even walking was hard for me. But this changed quickly. At first, my workouts were just long walks. Looking back, these long walks were moderately slow, but near the end, my dad prompted me to go slightly faster. After a while of doing this procedure, I was able to walk fast for the entire way. After a few months of doing this, I started running, walking, and jogging around the high-school jogging track. When the weather was cold, we could do these types of workouts at indoor tracks. Before my program ended, I was able to jog and run around the track eight times (2 miles) without stopping! I was never able to do even the 1-mile run before my program; I had obviously progressed during my program! I also used our treadmill many times for my workouts. It was hard for me, but I didn't mind because I would listen to music while doing this activity. Again, I followed the same procedure where I started out slow, and then increased my speed near the end.

I never did any weight lifting before I started my program. My uncle explained to me that it is not a good idea for small kids to get into weight training like older teenage kids. So my dad just bought some hand weights, and I used those a few nights a week as part of my workouts. Trying to lift weights that you can barely lift is definitely not the way to go. Instead, concentrate on lifting lighter weights; do as many as you can. The next time you do your curls, push yourself to do one or two more than previously.

Sometimes I would combine types of activities for my workouts, like lifting weights and doing the treadmill. After lifting, I would walk for a few minutes on the treadmill, and then lift weights again. These workouts really made me sweat.

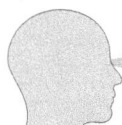

Check Your Understanding

1. **Why is it not a good idea to follow your instinctual urges in regard to the eating patterns of the hunter/gatherers?**

    Answer: *We are able to partake of a feast daily while this was not the case with the hunter/ gatherers.*

2. **What is the aspect of the Bases Loaded Program that is not in keeping with the ancient hunter/gatherer lifestyle?**

    Answer: *Nightly workouts are not in keeping with the ancient daytime hunt.*

3. **What advantage do those who do their workout at night have over those that do their workout in the morning hours?**

    Answer: *The late night workout offers many advantages. Workouts in the evening work better for a child's schedule. When we awake in the morning, there is no need to delay food. By eating early, we will be following the 12-hour eating cycle that the body naturally prefers. We will eat from sun to sun instead of noon to midnight. Since we will not be tired from a morning workout, we will have more energy during the day to study or work. At night exhaustion comes right before going to sleep rather than right after dinner. Best of all, we awake being a gram or two lighter, rather than the same weight we maintained for several years under the daylight plan.*

4. **Compare work-ins and workouts to a campfire.**

    Answer: *The burning bright flames of the campfire represent metabolism. We can compare small shavings and kindling to work-ins. The big logs can be compared to a workout.*

5. **Despite growing numbers of those doing workouts, what two instinctual urges contribute to America's obesity epidemic?**

    Answer: *Americans have forsaken an important instinctual urge (work-ins) and they are a little too zealous at following other instinctual urges (workout/eating patterns of the hunter/ gatherers).*

6. **Why is it important to vary your workouts?**

    Answer: *Exercise combinations are a lot like food combinations. Getting a variety of exercise helps to nourish the muscles of the body.*

7.   **Define work-ins.**

   Answer: *Work-ins are conscious and unconscious body movements that cause the metabolism to build in intensity.*

8.   **What is an easy way to remember the difference between a work-in and a workout?**

   Answer: *Work-ins keep the sweat "in" while workouts let the sweat "out" of the body.*

9.   **What are some examples of hunter/gatherer work-ins, and hunter/gatherer workouts?**

   Answer: *Examples of work-ins include, making traps, walking to the hunting grounds, gathering food items, or collecting firewood. Running after animals, or dragging a dead deer for a mile, are examples of a workout.*

10.   **What are some examples of modern day work-ins?**

   Answer: *A few examples of modern day work-ins include the fun physical activities, going for a walk, raking leaves, taking out the garbage, or walking up the stairs.*

11.   **Describe the Bases Loaded Program daily workout.**

   Answer: *The Bases Loaded workout occurs at the end of the evening shortly before retiring to bed. It lasts for 20-25 minutes. It starts slow and builds in intensity. The last few minutes of the workout or set of exercises is the most intense. Any exercise is acceptable as long as it causes one to breathe hard and sweat. Stretches should be done before and after the workout.*

12.   **Can we expect to lose weight if we fail to make work-ins and a workout part of the daily routine?**

   Answer: *No we must incorporate both work-ins and a workout into the daily routine in order to lose weight.*

Notes:

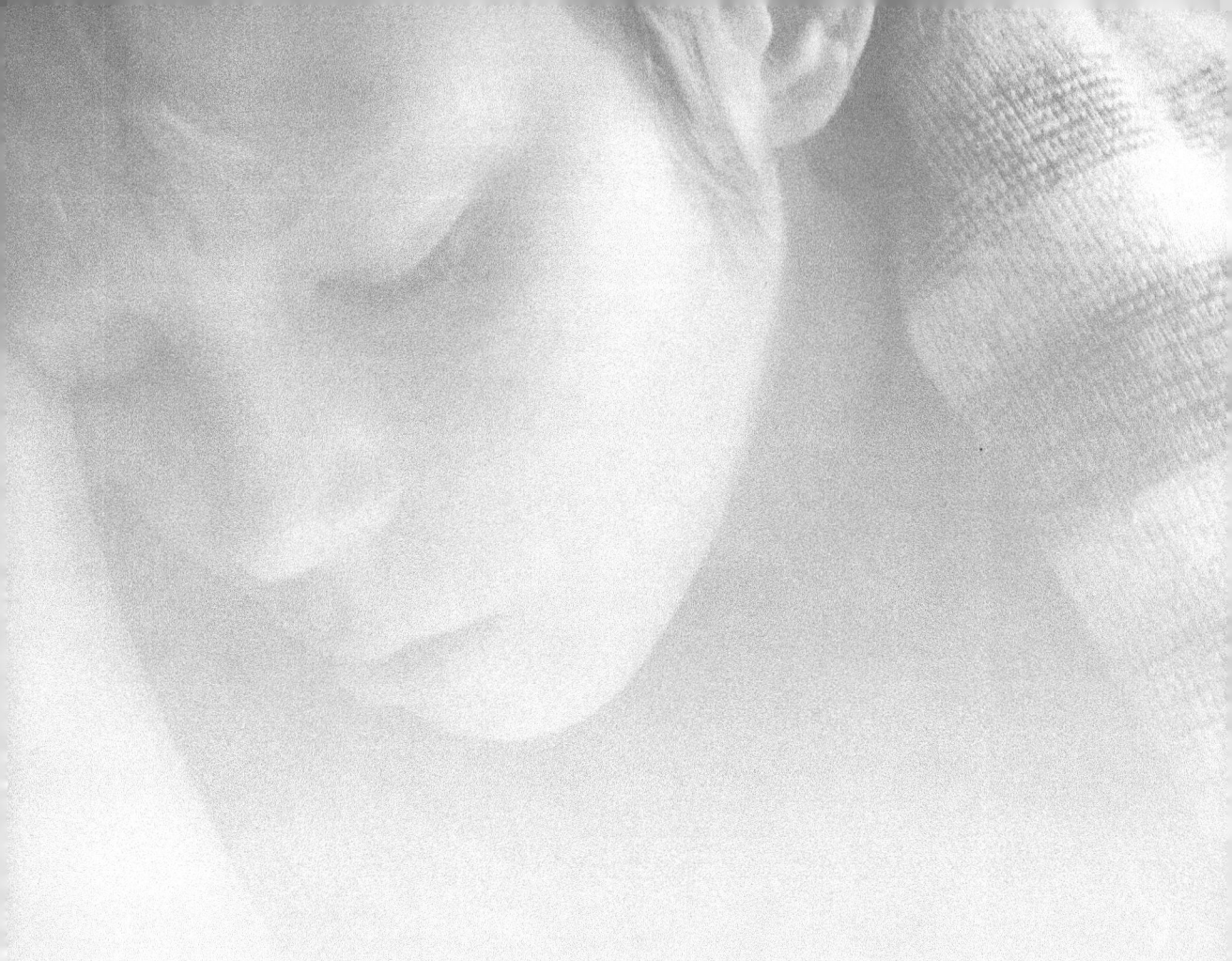

Proper rest is not only important for our physical health, but it is a vital part of our mental and emotional health.

Rest and Regeneration

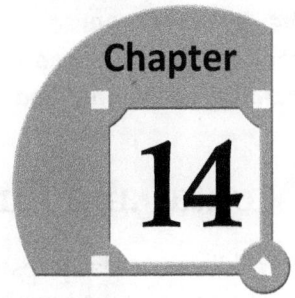

Chapter **14**

Sleep and rest play very powerful roles in the quest for ideal weight. One would think that staying awake longer would force the metabolism to work at a higher rate for a longer time. Naturally we would burn more energy and lose weight , but that is not the case.

I have found that the best way to understand metabolism, is to think of it as a person. That is why I sometimes refer to metabolism as, Mr. Metabolism. We all enjoy a good night of sleep. What happens when we do not get the needed rest? We move slowly through the day without much energy. We look forward to laying down on that bed so that we can enter the world of dreams.

Mr. Metabolism is no different. In fact, much of what we feel is actually the metabolism speaking to us. If we lack energy, it is because metabolism is conserving energy. When we get enough sleep and eat enough food in the morning, metabolism will work for us. We feel full of energy, and will be able do much in the way of mental and physical work.

Evidently, metabolism needs sufficient sleep time to erase the memory of the previous evening. Without enough sleep, metabolism's clock is a few hours off. It still believes that it is the evening of the previous day. Metabolism is still trying to get ready for a new day by slowing the body down to prepare it for sleep.

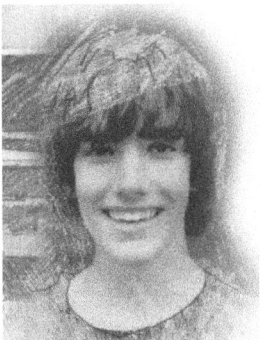

Rest is another important factor. It is crucial for weight loss. Doing a workout at the end of the night forces your metabolism to work hard. After you do a workout, it is quite easy to go to sleep. I can definitely say that the combination of getting a good workout, a good night's sleep, and a great breakfast helps me to do well in my studies.

Vacations are the greatest! Some of my best memories and funny stories come from our family vacations. Also, it is important for me to have one day of rest during the week where I try to rest from schoolwork. My favorite thing to do on my day of rest is to play the guitar and listen to music. Good music brings peace to my mind and definitely helps me be a better person. Make sure your kid gets plenty of rest at night and don't make them work all the time. Do fun things together during the week and on family vacations and don't forget to listen to good music!

Mental and Emotional Rest

In addition to daily rest, we need weekly and seasonal rest, as well. Pick one day a week to refrain from the evening workout. Go for a walk instead. My family chooses Sunday as the day of rest. If work schedules permit, go on a vacation in the summer time. Vacations help everyone in the family to get away from the daily stress. Vacations can sometimes be stressful, especially when one's family is large, but it is a different kind of stress. The fond memories that we create for the family during vacations far outweigh the stress. Proper rest is not only important for physical health, but it is a vital part of mental and emotional health. Seen in this light, proper rest coupled with workouts, help to recreate and regenerate the core of who we are. Who are we anyway?

"When beginning to work with a new patient I will frequently draw a large circle. Then at the circumference I will draw a small niche. Pointing to the inside of the niche, I say, 'That represents your conscious mind. All the rest of the circle, 95 percent or more, represents your unconscious.'" [64]

According to Scott Peck, the famous American psychiatrist, the conscious part of the mind is a truly small part of us. The larger part, or core part of us, lies within the unconscious and contains knowledge and truths that "await" re-remembering.

"The development of consciousness is the development of awareness in our conscious mind of knowledge along with our unconscious mind, which already possesses that knowledge. It is a process of the conscious mind coming into synchrony with the unconscious." [65]

Part of the growth that we as human beings go through in life is to promote this "synchrony" between the conscious and unconscious parts of us. As we do so, we can become extensions of our creator.

"Were we to become all unconscious, we would be indeed like the newborn infant, one with God but incapable of any action that might make the presence of God felt in the world." [66]

Healthy emotional and spiritual growth, then, requires a recognition and marriage of two complementary entities. The welding together of these two entities brings maturity and progression and helps us on the road that leads to happiness.

"The goal of theology presented here, and that of most mystics is exactly the opposite. It is not to become an ego-less, unconscious babe. Rather it is to develop a mature, conscious ego which then can become the ego of God." [67]

Rest and sleep, then, are necessary conditions, which allow the conscious to connect back to one's core and develop the marriage of the conscious and unconscious minds.

Power Within Us

Notice in the next visual **(Figure 35)** the hidden power of the Nourishment Triangle. The N-Triangle connects to a hidden circular shape that dominates the physical, mental and spiritual parts of us. Since this shape represents the type of rest we receive when we are asleep, it is shaded like the Nourishment Triangle. Just as we "receive" nourishment from food, so it is that we "receive" something from the period of deep sleep. Since "physical activity" is an act of giving out, the light shaded Physical Activity Triangle represents a small deviation from the overall daily scheme of receiving energy and rest.

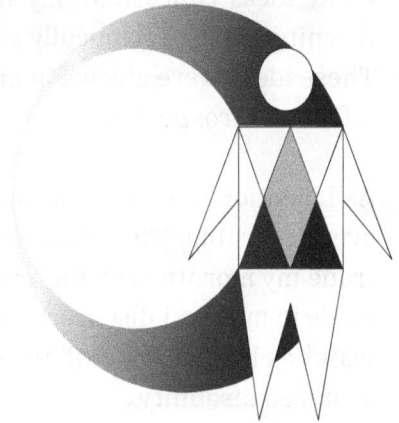

Figure 35: Hidden Power of the Nourishment Triangle - The Nourishment Triangle is connected to a dark shaded circle, which represents the nourishment that we receive to our subconscious when we sleep, meditate or pray.

With awareness of the power within us, let us re-evaluate the Nourishment Triangle. According to the configuration of the N-Triangle, the BL-Program values the morning hours for receiving food and rest. We have already discussed the subject of food. Now let us consider rest. If Scott Peck is right, and the unconscious, the larger part of us, is the God part of us, then it makes sense that we should devote some quality time, besides sleep, to this important part of us. It also makes sense that this time should be in the morning, when dreams from the unconscious are still on the surface, when we can retrieve them before the rush of the conscious world buries them.

Rest, then, is that period of "conscious" time where we open ourselves to the "hidden" part of us. Since the Bases Loaded Program has us refrain from a five-mile jog first thing in the morning, let us devote this time instead to a morning walk. After breakfast, when the children are off to school, take the baby or pet dog for a walk. We can pray or meditate during this time. We can use this time to clear the mind and ponder the bigger picture. Going for a walk, especially on sunny days, allows light to enter the body through the eyes. Research has found that sunlight increases metabolism and has many other therapeutic qualities.

"To our metabolism, spending the day indoors is virtually the same as spending the day in darkness. It stimulates the inherent physiological processes associated with sleeping and gaining weight." [68]

I have found that the morning hours are the most creative hours of the day. I have had many ideas concerning my family, or my profession, come into my mind during early morning walks. Technically speaking, these thoughts did not actually come into my mind. These ideas were always in my mind. I happened to discover them through my conscious effort of introspection.

As I mentioned earlier, I have always enjoyed workouts. For many years, I ran a few miles every morning. That changed when I developed arthritis in my left knee. I decided to trade my morning run for a morning walk. I cannot begin to express the difference it has made in my life. I discovered many of the ideas contained in this book during my morning walks as I pondered both the problems Joe faced, and the problems I faced with my newly acquired disability.

Encourage your child to have some quiet time during the weekend and summer break. When driving them to school or while they are eating breakfast, ask your children about their dreams during the night. Parents can gain many insights from the dreams of their children.

I believe that Scott Peck is right. The answers to all challenges and problems are within us waiting to be rediscovered. This rediscovery, then, requires getting a good night of sleep. I trust that parents know their own body and their child's body well enough to determine what constitutes a good sleep. For me, it is seven hours, for Joe it is nine hours. Get a good night of sleep after your workout, and dream dreams. Ponder these dreams, or even write them down when first awakening. Give it a try, walk, do not run, and have a little quiet time after breakfast. It is amazing all that we hear, and all that we do not hear if we take the time to listen within.

Troubleshooting Your Child's Program

When we speak of troubleshooting, we speak of adjustments "towards" the Bases Loaded Program as opposed to "away" from it.

Since it is not possible to monitor your child all day, sometimes they may veer slightly from the principles contained in this book. This section will help the family if things are not going quite right. Take advantage of your quiet time to troubleshoot any problems concerning the Bases Loaded Program. I realize that some parents do not have the luxury of a morning walk or quiet time in the morning. Perhaps, there is one day a week, where the work schedule is open. If that is the case, please treat yourself to a space of time, preferably in the morning that is just for meditation.

Parents have the power within themselves to solve challenges that may arise concerning their child's program. Follow correct principles, heed any special advice that your family doctor gives, and listen within for inspiration concerning details or issues that are specific to your child. While I cannot give specific advice concerning your child, I can offer some general guidelines concerning troubleshooting.

First guideline: Be patient in troubleshooting. Remember, the Bases Loaded Program is not a quick fix program. As stated in the introduction of this book, the physical changes that Joe went through in the course of a year's time were imperceptible to those who lived with Joe on a day-to-day basis. Society has conditioned us to expect results quickly, but as a parent and coach, do not be like society. Whenever making an adjustment to your child's program, continue for a week or two before making another adjustment. Because the physical changes are so imperceptible, it takes time to assess the adjustments.

Second: Be aware of Mr. Metabolism's long-term memory, especially in the initial stages of your child's program. If your child is not losing weight, or if their weight seems to be in a holding pattern, it could be that their body has been in "partial starvation mode," and is holding on to some deficient nutrients. Continue to follow the program and eat nutritiously. Your child's body will adjust accordingly. The first victory in the BL- Program is to slow down and halt the excessive weight gain that burdens your child. Once that has happened, then, we can start reversing the process and work on losing fat.

Third: Always remember and compare "Obesity's Game Plan" and the "Bases Loaded Game Plan." Most weight management issues connect to the battle between these opposing plans. Obesity wants us to be in starvation mode all day and night. The BL-Plan avoids starvation mode during the waking hours. The best feedback that a parent will receive from their child concerning the program is an answer to a simple question that the parent should ask periodically before dinner. The question is this; "How do you feel?" If your child is incorporating the principles of the BL-Program correctly, the answer to that question would be, "fine," or "okay." If the answer is, "starved" or "tired," then there is room for concern. The BL-Plan avoids starvation mode during the waking hours, by following the natural 12-hour cycle of eating from sunrise to sunset. The response "I'm hungry" could mean that your child just needs a snack, but look closer and make sure that your child follows correct principles.

Fourth: Make sure your child is following the principles connected to the Physical Activity Triangle and the Nourishment Triangle. The heads of those triangles are just as powerful as their bases, or the wide part of the triangle. Let us consider the Nourishment Triangle first. If your child is respecting the natural 12 hour cycles, eating nutritious food, getting their supplements and enough rest, but still cannot lose half a pound a week, it could be that your child is getting too much food for dinner. Not wanting to have physical fun after dinner, could be an indication that this is the problem. To solve this problem, do not reduce the amount of food your child receives during the whole day. Just move some of the food from dinner to breakfast or lunch, thus creating a smaller dinner. In other words, keep the head of the N-Triangle sharp and pointed up. The head of the Physical Activity Triangle also needs to be sharp but pointed down. In other words, work-ins, low and moderate physical activities occupy the morning and afternoon hours. Fun activities and a workout occupy the early evening and late night respectively.

On the other hand, if your child feels too tired to do anything after dinner it could be that they are too tired from physical activities at school. In a recent study, researchers measured the amount of movement and physical activity experienced by three different sets of school children. One set experienced vigorous physical activity, another set experienced moderate physical activity, and the last set experienced low physical activity during the school day hours. The researches continued to monitor the children after school. Here is what they found.

"And no matter how much PE they got during school hours, when you look at the whole day, the kids from the three schools moved the same amount, at about the same intensity. The kids at the fancy private school underwent significantly more physical activity before 3 p.m., but overall they didn't move more."[69]

In terms of the Physical Activity Triangle size and orientation, what does this research indicate? Considering the physical activities and movements of school age children for the whole day, their PA-Triangles are the same size or present the same amount of light shaded surface area. The only thing that varies are the orientations. Some point up (significant activity at school), and some point down (moderate and low activity at school).

"Once they get home if they are very active in school, they are probably staying still a bit more because they've already expended so much energy,"" says Alissa Fre'meaux, a biostatistician who helped conduct the study. ""The others are more likely to grab a bike and run around after school."[70]

In plain language, children only have so much energy to expend during the course of their waking hours. If they expend too much energy at school, then they will lack energy in the evening. If they experience rigorous physical activity at school, and combine this activity with sparse amounts of food rather than the bulk of their calories for the day, then they will feel exhausted in the late afternoon, making it hard to perform any physical task. As we discussed earlier in the book, these conditions lead to overeating in the evening hours when metabolism slows down to conservation mode, which in turn causes weight gain.

If your child is experiencing vigorous physical activity at school that causes them to sweat and get out of breath, switch your child to a PE class that is less strenuous. If this is not possible, consider getting a medical exemption from your family doctor that would limit your child to low and moderate physical activities during the day. If successful, make sure your child follows the BL-Program by doing a good workout at the end of the evening.

Troubleshooting Your Own Program

Parents having trouble losing half a pound a week, after the first few weeks of the program, should follow the same four guidelines listed above. Things will be slightly different for a parent when it comes to sharpening the head of the Physical Activity Triangle. If your job involves hard physical work during the day (PA-Triangle pointed up), avoid the pitfall of refueling exclusively at night. Get the bulk of your calories at breakfast and lunch. Make dinner a light meal. Participate in the fun physical activities of the evening. When your child does a workout, do a work-in.

If your job involves sitting around most of the day (PA-Triangle pointed down), it could mean that the head of your Physical Activities Triangle, the sharp portion that is pointing downward, is cut off. As explained earlier, we need to figure out creative ways to incorporate hourly work-ins during the day. Include your boss or manager in this process. Loan them this book, or buy your employer a copy and present it as a gift. A smart employer or manager will see the benefits to the business that hourly work-ins will bring. I am confident that they will truly work for the good of the company if they understand the principles contained in this book.

Sharpening the Nourishment Triangle may be more challenging for adults than children. Maybe it is habit, but adults seem to reward themselves with a large dinner at the end of a hard day of work. I was no different from the majority of adult Americans. I found that sharpening the N-Triangle played a big part in my own program to achieve ideal weight.

Before the Bases Loaded Program, I tried to stay physically fit by exercising daily. I ate well and took daily supplements. I tried to get proper rest. The ideal weight for my age and height is about 205 pounds. All things considered I did pretty well keeping my weight to 215 pounds. For some reason, I could not get that last 10 pounds of fat off! Since I was living a fairly healthy lifestyle, the changes I incorporated through the Bases Loaded Program did not seem that drastic. I changed my workout times to the end of the evening. I incorporated more work-ins during the morning, afternoon, and early evening hours. I adjusted my eating cycle. Still that extra 10 pounds of fat would not go away from my body.

Finally, I pushed dinner to an earlier time. I began having a late lunch or early dinner at 2:00 or 3:00 p.m. The last food of the evening for me came between 5:00-6:30 p.m. It was always small and nutritious. Several times it was no more than a salad or an antioxidant shake, but I always felt satisfied since I received the bulk of my daily food earlier in the day. This final adjustment made the difference. I lost the 10 pounds of fat and achieved my ideal weight within 5 months.

Evolution v. Creationism

Here are some thoughts that came to me on a morning walk. I realize that writing about this subject may seem strange to some reading this book. What does this "150 year old" debate have to do with childhood obesity? The answer is rather simple. If indeed a benevolent creator, programmed the human body, then logically the creator desires to help us overcome obstacles in life. Knowing that we have a benevolent programmer gives us confidence in early morning meditations or prayers, that solutions will come to mind concerning the program. With this, I would like to offer my opinion concerning these two theories.

I believe that God created man and woman, but in doing so, the programmer used the hunter/gatherers as prototypes. Biologically we are almost identical to them. Spiritually, intellectually and in terms of outward "image" we are patterned after God. If the theory I explained is correct, the earliest hunter/gatherers would not be true ancestors, but rather "step ancestors." Such a theory would explain the huge intelligence gap that separates human beings from the earliest "human like" creatures. It would also explain the biological linkage to hunter/gatherers of old. Questions arise from this theory that I have just explained. If human beings are indeed "programmed" by the hand of a benevolent creator, why then are we biologically patterned after the hunter/gatherers? Why is metabolism programmed the way it is with "limited memory" and starvation mode?

Why Starvation Mode and Limited Memory?

Here we are again, back to the same question we pondered earlier. Now there is a different aspect to consider. If my theory is correct, then surely the programmer foresaw the day when human beings would not have to spend all their time and energy looking for food, as was the case with the hunter/gatherers. Should not the metabolism be programmed with a more sophisticated memory, one that could take inventory of the "extra fuel" or fat cells held in reserve? I believe the key to answering this question requires an expanded understanding of the spiritual aspect regarding the human family. Were we sent to this earth as part of a contest, to see which individuals, through their intellect, cunning, and social bonding, could grab the biggest piece of "economic" and "temporal" pie?

I believe that there is a higher purpose for human creation. We are not "islands" unto ourselves. We are here to become "all" that we can be; intellectually, spiritually, physically, emotionally, and socially. If that is the case, it makes sense that programming "starvation mode" and metabolism's "limited memory" into human beings, helps us achieve the full measure of creation. A full analysis of how these programmed elements help us develop intellectually, spiritually, emotionally and socially, might prove interesting to many readers, but it would require several chapters of writing to do so. Suffice it to say, all aspects of human development necessitate time and physical survival. How can a person develop fully emotionally or socially if starvation claims their life while they are young? Couple the above thought, with the knowledge that three fourths of the world's population is considered "third world," and we can begin to see why we are programmed the way that we are. It is hard for most of us, in the developed nations of the world, to imagine a life where "death from starvation" is a daily concern. The threat of starvation is still the rule, rather than the exception, for the vast majority of the human family.

When we ponder this situation long enough, the realization of something quite profound comes to mind. The "Benevolent Programmer" is truly benevolent. "Starvation mode" and metabolism's "limited memory" are great gifts. They are great gifts given to each and every person born into this world, to ensure their physical survival. Regardless of race, gender, or ethnic background, the programmer treats us with equal respect and love. God desires that each of us might live so that we can become all that we can become!

The Parable of the Wise Father

There was a parent with four children. The four children were two sets of twins, two girls and two boys born within two consecutive years. The father worked with dedication and love, to provide his children with all the necessities of life. Over time, the father amassed a great fortune. He had the power to provide not only the needs, but also the "wants" of his children. The father acted with prudence, though, and did not indulge his children with everything they wanted. He did not want to spoil his children with "things," but rather encouraged them to work and study hard, help each other, and learn the true meaning of happiness.

The time came when the children grew to maturity, and each went off to a different university. The father pondered the best way to provide for his children now that they were on their own. He could give them a credit card and allow them to get whatever they wanted, whenever they wanted. Such a method, though, seemed to contradict everything that he taught his children growing up. After much thought, he decided to set up a "low activity bank account" in the respective city where each child lived.

These accounts were like the account that the father created for his struggling business years ago. Each child would be given enough money to provide for their schooling needs but no more. He reasoned that such an account would help his children to manage and budget their money wisely. Instead of getting everything that they wanted, they would have to be wise stewards. The father proved to be wise in his reasoning. The bank accounts encouraged his children to develop qualities of thrift and responsibility. The accounts also encouraged the children to help one another and to communicate with their father.

Quite often the aging father received phone calls from his children seeking advice or expressing gratitude. In all of these communications, the father felt great joy.

The meaning of the parable is perhaps obvious. The father represents the "Benevolent Programmer," the low activity bank account represents the gifts of "starvation mode" and metabolism's "limited memory." The fruits of these gifts are the virtuous qualities engendered within the children. The "communication" between the father and his children represents meditation and prayer.

Okay! A Few More From the Funny Book

May 2007 (Joe 13 years old) I told Joe today that I was "playing catch up" all day. Joe said, "Well, I eat catsup every day!"

May 2007 Joe sings, "Stir Fry, don't bother me, Stir Fry don't bother me, Stir Fry don't bother me, or I will gobble some body!"

Feb. 2008 (Joe 14 years old)
Joe was writing an essay on Henry V & Sir Thomas Moore, and wrote; ". . . or, we are just ponds in God's universal game of chess!" He meant "pawns," but we laughed so hard we almost died.

April 2009 (Joe 15 years old)
On a practice exam, Joe writes about "The Odyssey; " "In ancient Greece, a pheasant could become rich and powerful, but he was still considered a pheasant."

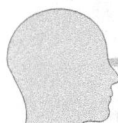

Check Your Understanding

1. **Is it true that staying awake longer forces the metabolism to work harder and thus helps us to lose weight?**

    Answer: *Not getting enough sleep causes the metabolism to go into conservation mode, so we will gain weight from lack of sleep.*

2. **If we fail to get enough sleep, will the metabolism be able to erase its memory and begin a new day?**

    Answer: *Metabolism is not able to erase its memory, which causes metabolism's clock to be a few hours off. At the start of a new day, metabolism is living in the past, still trying to prepare for sleep.*

3. **In addition to physical rest, what other type of rest do human beings need?**

    Answer: *Human beings need mental, emotional and spiritual rest.*

4. **Which part of the mind constitutes the "dominant" part of the mind; the conscious or unconscious?**

    Answer: *The unconscious mind constitutes the dominant part of us.*

5. **In troubleshooting a program, what part of the PA-Triangle or N-Triangle usually needs attention, the base or head?**

    Answer: *Troubleshooting a program usually involves fixing the head of one of the triangles.*

6. **Where and when can we find the answers to life's challenges?**

    Answer: *We can expect to find the answers to life's challenges within ourselves as we meditate or pray during the early morning hours.*

Unscientific as it may sound, love is the foundation principle of all the principles contained in Bases Loaded. To love and to be loved, that is the reason Bases Loaded works best when there are at least two involved.

OBESITY PUZZLE

CHILDHOOD   OBESITY

Getting Started and Finishing

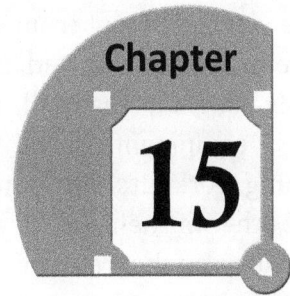

Having read to this point in the book, you have already taken the first step in a journey that hopefully will last a lifetime. You have read the theory behind Bases Loaded. You understand the working model and have seen the results. Now you want to incorporate the principles of this book into your own life. What is your next step?

Commitment

As discussed in the introduction, Bases Loaded is about achieving ideal weight within the setting of the family. If you are a family of one, and desire to incorporate the principles of the Bases Loaded Program into your life, then proceed to the next step. If you are a parent reading this book, then you will want to present this book to your child. Depending on the age and maturity of your child, you may have them read it, or show the pictures and explain the concepts to them. Bases Loaded is about making positive changes in life. Having read this book, you realize that in order for this program to work it requires effort by all involved. Understand the commitment, you must have to support your child in this program. Your child will have the courage to change if they see that same commitment to change within you, the parent.

Doctor, Equipment, Pictures, Scale

When everyone commits to the Bases Loaded Program, the next step is to visit your family pediatrician for an exam. It is a good idea to consult your family doctor, even if you do not think your child's weight issues are serious. Your pediatrician can help determine an appropriate weight for your child to achieve. Parents, when was the last time you had a checkup? We strongly recommend that you consult your doctor before starting this program, as well. Your doctor will be able to consult with you on the matters we have discussed in this book. Perhaps they will offer certain modifications that are right for you.

Once you have input from your doctors, there are just a few more preliminary things to do before getting started. Equipment needs will vary according to your child's needs. My family bought a treadmill, some hand weights, and a bench for lifting weights. These two sets of equipment proved to be invaluable since they added convenient options to the evening workouts. The equipment did not take up much room, and they complemented each other in their use. In many workouts, Joe and I rotated positions so that we would take turns on the treadmill while the other person lifted weights. If you do get a treadmill, buy the kind that has variable speeds that you can adjust manually. This will allow you to walk and run in patterns that you decide rather than being locked into a predetermined program. The set of hand weights only went to 20 pounds, so it was minimal in terms of cost.

Another useful tool is that of a strong light. I am referring to the natural lights people buy to relieve wintertime depression. It is evident that light is the main catalyst for setting the time clock that governs metabolism. The presence of light increases metabolism intensity, while the absence of light decreases metabolism to conservation mode. If you live in a section of the country where the sun hides a part of the year, this tool will help increase your metabolism on those overcast days.

With the equipment needs set in order, grab a camera and take some "before" photos, to keep a visual record of your child's weight loss. Take pictures, but put them in a drawer to be pulled out in 6 months. We want these "before" shots to be viewed, only after your child has lost 15 or 20 pounds. After your child loses 15 or 20 pounds, pull out the old photos and take some more pictures. Viewing weight loss by contrasting these later photos to the earlier photos will then become a means to inspire and encourage your child.

Buy an inexpensive scale, and keep a record of the weight loss for all program participants. Weigh yourself and your child once a week, no more, no less. Remember this is not a quick fix. Ideal weight will be accomplished in months, not days, so be patient about it. Do not check your child's weight every day. Make sure this weighing happens first thing in the morning before eating or drinking anything. Designate a weigh day, preferably in the middle of the week, so that the weekly weighing occurs under consistent circumstances. Keep a simple record of the weekly weighing, along with pertinent notes **(Figure 36)**.

Fat Calibration Test

Get a fat calibration test done for your child. Consult with your doctor or local fitness center as to, where one can get a test done. The most accurate fat calibration test uses a fat calibration pod. A fat calibration pod looks like a little rocket ship capsule. The person receiving the test gets into a bathing suit outfit and simply sits in the pod. Joe tested at a local university, and the cost was about ten dollars. The test generates a printout **(Figure 37)** that breaks down body mass into lean muscle versus fat. Knowing this information will help in the future, when your child has attained their goal of ideal weight. A second fat calibration test should be given when your child achieves ideal weight. Let us view and discuss Joe's calibration measurements.

Knowing the Finish Line

Notice **(Figure 36)** that Joe achieved his goal of ideal weight Sept. 9, 2006. At that point, we should have had Joe get another fat calibration test. We had previously planned to have the

Joe's Weight Chart		
Date	**Weight**	**Notes**
10/01/05	142.5	
10/13/05	137.7	Calibration weight
11/01/05	142.5	
12/03/05	141.0	Lost 1.5 pounds Nov.
12/08/05	143.0	Highest weight of program
12/15/05	142.0	
12/17/05	141.0	
12/23/05	140.0	
01/06/06	137.5	Lost 5 pounds Dec.
01/15/06	138.5	Gain 1.5 lbs.
01/22/06	135.0	
02/01/06	131.5	Lost 6 pounds Jan.
02/11/06	134.5	Gained 3 lbs.
03/12/06	131.0	Lost .5 pounds Feb.
04/01/06	130.5	Lost .5 lbs. March
04/10/06	129.5	
05/02/11	129.0	Lost 1.5 pounds April
05/25/06	127.0	
06/01/06	125.5	Lost 3.5 pounds May
06/01/06	125.5	
06/04/06	124.0	
06/10/06	125.5	

Figure 36: Joe's Weight Chart - Keep a record of weight loss/gain. This helps assess the effectiveness of the program.

second test performed on his one-year calibration anniversary, which was still a month away. In the next few weeks, Joe worked himself very hard. Instead of losing half a pound per week, he was losing over twice that amount. We decided to have the fat calibration test 11 days early, on Oct. 2, 2006.

Compare the "lean body weight" of the two calibration tests. Notice that Joe lost one pound of muscle mass. In retrospect, I think Joe lost this one pound of muscle during the last month of his program due to protein catabolism. Herein we see why bodybuilders routinely get fat calibration tests to monitor their lean body weight. With these tests, they are able to make adjustments to their program to prevent muscle loss from becoming a serious problem.

In the BL-Program, the first test gives you a benchmark for your lean body weight. With the second calibration test, one can compare the lean body weight at the end of the program to the benchmark weight. In your child's program, if their second test shows that muscle weight improves, you might consider continuing their program for another week, whereupon you would get another calibration test. You would continue this close weekly monitoring until there was no change in the muscle mass, or you notice a retrograde in

Joe's Weight Chart Continued		
Date	**Weight**	**Notes**
07/03/06	120.0	Lost 5.5 pounds June
07/12/06	118.0	
07/23/06	115.0	Lost 3 pounds scout camp
07/26/06	113.0	Lost 30 pounds from December 8th
08/02/06	113.5	Lost 6.5 pounds July
08/05/06	112.5	
08/23/06	110.0	
09/04/06	107.5	Lost 6 pounds August
09/09/06	108.0	*Ideal weight – Took pictures
09/18/06	106.0	
10/02/06	103.7	Calibration weight – Lost 4 pounds Sept. Lost a pound of muscle
		over program; trainer says it's normal.
10/08/06	103.0	Lost 40 pounds from Dec. 8

Figure 36 Continued: Joe's Weight Chart - Keep a record of weight loss/gain. This helps assess the effectiveness of the program.

Fat Calibration Records (2005-2006)

Body Composition Analysis			
Name:	Joe Cassler	Date:	10/13/05
Age:	11	Height:	61 ins (155 cms)
Gender:	M	Model:	Siri 1961
Technician	KS	Density	1.000 kg/l
Percent Fat	44.8 %	Fat Weight	61.7 lbs
Percent Lean	55.2 %	Lean Weight	76.0 lbs
		Total Weight	137.7 lbs

Body Composition Analysis			
Name:	Joe Cassler	Date:	10/02/06
Age:	12	Height:	63 ins (160 cms)
Gender:	M	Model:	Siri 1961
Technician	CT	Density	1.036 kg/l
Percent Fat	27.6 %	Fat Weight	28.7 lbs
Percent Lean	72.4 %	Lean Weight	75.0 lbs
		Total Weight	103.7 lbs

Figure 37: Body Composition Analysis or Fat Calibration - It is important to keep records of your child's lean weight, to make sure that the weight loss is fat, rather than muscle.

the muscle mass. Once muscle mass has plateaued or starts to recede, then your child has officially completed the Bases Loaded Program.

It is extremely important that your child stop the nightly workouts if you discover any loss or retrograde of muscle mass. The best thing they can do to stop the process of protein catabolism is to relax. Have your child stop working so hard, and make sure they get plenty of protein in their diet.

Cooling Down the Program

We officially ended Joe's program by celebrating his accomplishment with a party, but not much changed in Joe's life after that. Joe maintained an active lifestyle, going on walks and doing fun physical activities. Eventually, Joe resumed his workouts on his own, doing a few workouts a week instead of six. We continued to check his lean muscle mass with periodic fat calibration tests **(Figure 38)**. Comparing the results of these tests, notice that Joe's lean muscle mass increased over the course of a year. During the same period, his body fat weight stayed below 24 percent. Joe's body was changing, and it was a change in the right direction. The greatest aspect of this new direction was the fact that Joe was in charge of the change. As a parent, the most rewarding moment of the Base's Loaded Program comes with the realization that your child has gained control of their own body and that they in a sense can be "given the car keys." They do not need to be taught how to drive any longer. The principles have become second nature to them, a part of their life!

Adjusting the Body's Schedule

Now that, the preliminaries are out of the way, and you have the big picture, you can get to work, or should I say, you can start having family fun. Realize that the hardest part might already be over. The hardest part of the battle is committing to do the program! The only real tricky part happens in the first 24 hours, when your family starts to live the principles set forth in this book. Shifting the body's eating habits back to their normal cycle is comparable to getting over jet lag. Some people are probably thinking, "How in the world am I going to start eating food in the waking hours, my body is not used to that!"

Here is what I suggest. Your family should begin this program on a chosen day, at "dinner time." Go through your regular morning rituals on that day. Let all involved know, let it be written on the calendar, such and such a day, the family fun begins. Eat a modest dinner. After dinner have physical fun, and do a workout at the end of the evening. Go to bed a little earlier, so that everyone might wake a little earlier. Now that, everyone has gone 12 hours without food, they should be hungry. Since they are up a little earlier than usual, they have time to eat. So eat! Your family's adjustment into the Bases Loaded Program has been successful.

Secret of True Transformation

Here are a few more thoughts about getting started. If your child has a few favorite junk food snacks still left in the pantry upon starting the program, do not throw away the items. Your child will get upset and think that you are fanatical, not a good way to have family fun. Just let these snacks run out, and resolve never to buy them again. Eventually, replace all the old snacks with wholesome food. Try this experiment. Put the old snacks on the snack table along with the nuts and celery. If your child is like Joe, an amazing thing will happen. Their first preference will be the old snacks, but you will also find that your child will eat the corn chips and bean dip, or carrots and low fat ranch dip. When the old snacks run out after a few days, your child will supplement the good snacks with more good snacks and will hardly complain about the loss of the old snacks.

Body Composition Analysis			
Name:	Joseph Cassler	**Date:**	01/10/07
Age:	12	**Height:**	63 ins (160 cms)
Gender:	M	**Model:**	Siri 1961
Technician	AB	**Density**	1.045 kg/l
Percent Fat	23.5 %	**Fat Weight**	23.7 lbs
Percent Lean	76.5 %	**Lean Weight**	77.1 lbs
		Total Weight	100.9 lbs

Body Composition Analysis			
Name:	Joseph Cassler	**Date:**	06/05/07
Age:	13	**Height:**	64 ins (163 cms)
Gender:	M	**Model:**	Siri 1961
Technician	JR	**Density**	1.045 kg/l
Percent Fat	20.8 %	**Fat Weight**	21.2 lbs
Percent Lean	79.2 %	**Lean Weight**	80.9 lbs
		Total Weight	102.2 lbs

Figure 38: More Calibration Records - Continue to chart your child's lean body weight after the program.

Body Composition Analysis			
Name:	Joe Cassler	Date:	10/25/07
Age:	12	Height:	64 ins (163 cms)
Gender:	M	Model:	Siri 1961
Technician	JR	Density	1.045 kg/l
Percent Fat	23.8 %	Fat Weight	25.4 lbs
Percent Lean	76.2 %	Lean Weight	81.3 lbs
		Total Weight	106.7 lbs

Figure 38 Continued: More Calibration Records - Continue to chart your child's lean body weight after the program.

The above real life observation gives us interesting insight into two related topics, convenience and comfort. We sometimes call junk food "convenience food," but who is it convenient for? The above observation shows that Joe was able to replace junk food with wholesome food, as long as it was convenient. The reason we call junk food convenience food, has to do with us adults who get the food. When we buy convenience food for the family, us parents involvement with that food is minimal. Perhaps we eat some of it ourselves, but we do not prepare or make the food. It is all prepared, processed and packaged, for the convenience of us busy parents.

We also refer to junk food as "comfort food." In my home, we have comfort food, but it is not junk food. In my home, everyone knows that if someone is sick, Dad will make his famous mashed potatoes and healthy gravy. Without fail, my potatoes make the family member feel better for some magical reason. Come to think of it, there is a sort of magic involved. You might have figured out what I am suggesting. I often tell my family after serving them a snack or a meal, "I made it with love." I believe that love is the magical quality that transforms my mashed potatoes and gravy, and other dishes, into comfort food, or soul food as my wife calls it. Unscientific as it may sound, love is the foundation principle of all the principles contained in Bases Loaded. To love and be loved, that is the reason Bases Loaded works best when there are at least two involved.

What is the message a child receives when their parent takes the time to prepare wholesome snacks for them? What message does a parent send when they play catch, or go on a bike ride with their child after dinner? The message can be worded many ways; "They care about me," "They sacrifice for me," "They like me," or "They think I am worthwhile." In the end, all of these messages have their origin in the very real transforming power we call love. Love is the transforming power behind Bases Loaded. Love is the reason you read this book, and it should be your guide and companion as you implement these principles into the lives of your family.

A Daily Schedule

The Metabolism Hour Glass **(Figure 39)** provides us with a basic daily schedule that will guide us during the Bases Loaded Program. Notice that the day begins at the bottom and builds upward. By now, it is probably obvious that the ideal shape for the Metabolism Diamond is an hourglass. Incorporating this simple master plan into family life, will bring health, energy, and vitality to the lives of family members. Following the Bases Loaded Master Plan rids children of the burdens obesity places on them. Over time, they will be able to focus their full faculties to school work, developing their talents, and pursuing their interests. This, in turn, will help them reach their physical, intellectual, and emotional potentials.

The Metabolism Hour Glass

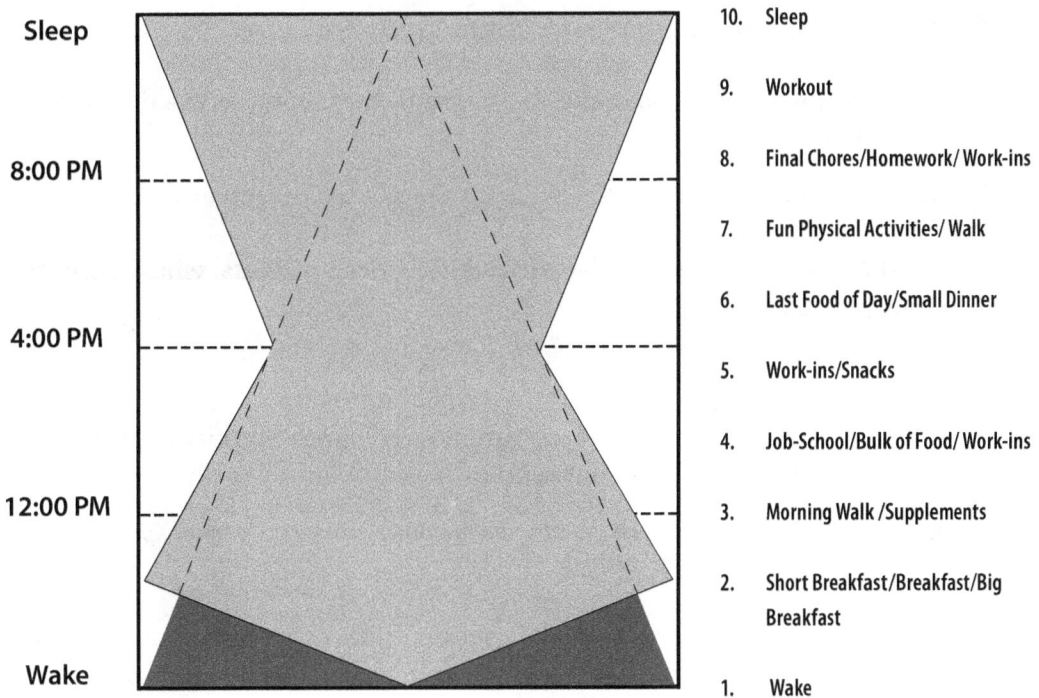

Figure 39: The Metabolism Hour Glass - The ideal shape that we want our metabolism to follow in the course of a day, as seen here, is wide at the bottom and wide at the top. The shape is similar to an hour glass and is obtained by following the schedule enumerated along the side. Following this simple master plan will bring energy and vitality to the lives of our family, and will allow our children to develop their talents and reach towards their full potentials.

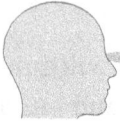

✔ Check Your Understanding

1.　**What are the four principles that comprise the Food Cornerstone?**

　　Answer: *The four principles comprising the Food Cornerstone are; Eat a Variety of Food, Avoid Junk Food, Replace Quick Release Energy Foods with Slow Release Energy Foods, and Replace Bad Fats with Good Fats.*

2.　**What is the name of the index we use to gauge "energy release" foods?**

　　Answer: *The Glycemic Index gauges the energy release (slow/fast) of specific food items.*

3.　**What is the name of the supplement that protects the body from heavy metal poisoning?**

　　Answer: *Glutathione protects the body from heavy metal poisoning.*

4.　**What is the name, used in the BL-Program, that refers to the time from sunrise to sunset?**

　　Answer: *The Natural Eating Cycle refers to the time from sunrise to sunset.*

5.　**What are some of the positive attitudes children possess, which parents should emulate?**

　　Answer: *We should have physical fun and learn to "eat to work" rather than "work to eat."*

6.　**What two aspects of the BL-Program, are the contemporary counterparts of the hunter/gatherers, "preparation of the hunt" and the "hunt?"**

　　Answer: *Work-ins and workouts are the contemporary counterparts to the "preparation of the hunt" and the "hunt" respectively.*

7.　**Is it true that modern research has shown that collectively, the amount of physical movement children accomplish in the course of a day is consistent, and it is only the time at which they accomplish these movements that varies?**

　　Answer: *True, amount of physical movement children accomplish in the course of a day is consistent in terms of length and intensity. Only the time of the day that these activities occur vary.*

8. **Explain the previous question in terms of the Physical Activities Triangle.**

Answer: *From recent research, we can conclude that the surface area of the Physical Activities Triangle does not vary from child to child. It is the orientation of the triangles that vary. Some triangles point up, and others point down.*

9. **Why is it so important to have a fat calibration test done before and at the end of the Bases Loaded Program?**

Answer: *Fat calibration tests are a critical part of the Bases Loaded Program. These tests guard program participants against the "unseen enemy" of protein catabolism. The first test gives us a "benchmark" of the lean muscle mass versus the fat mass. The last test determines the program's finish line.*

10. **When is the BL-Program officially finished?**

Answer: *We finish the program when we achieve ideal weight, and calibration tests indicate that lean muscle weight is the same as the benchmark muscle weight.*

11. **What circumstances would merit a continuation of the program, and at what point does the program end?**

Answer: *If the second calibration test indicates an increase in muscle mass, the program can continue as long as the parent monitors the child's muscle mass with weekly calibration tests. Celebrate the end of the program when the calibration test shows that the muscle weight has plateaued or retrograded.*

12. **What is the phrase, that best captures the secret of true transformation?**

Answer: *"To love and be loved" is the phrase that best describes the secret of true transformation.*

CONCLUSION:

SEDIMENTARY LIFESTYLE

DIETING

REFINED
CARBS

IMPROPER
FASTING

JUNK
FOOD

BAD FATS

BINGE

OBESITY

Fastballs
Curveballs
Change-ups

CHILDHOOD

OBESITY

CATCHER
Discouragement
Hopelessness
Failure

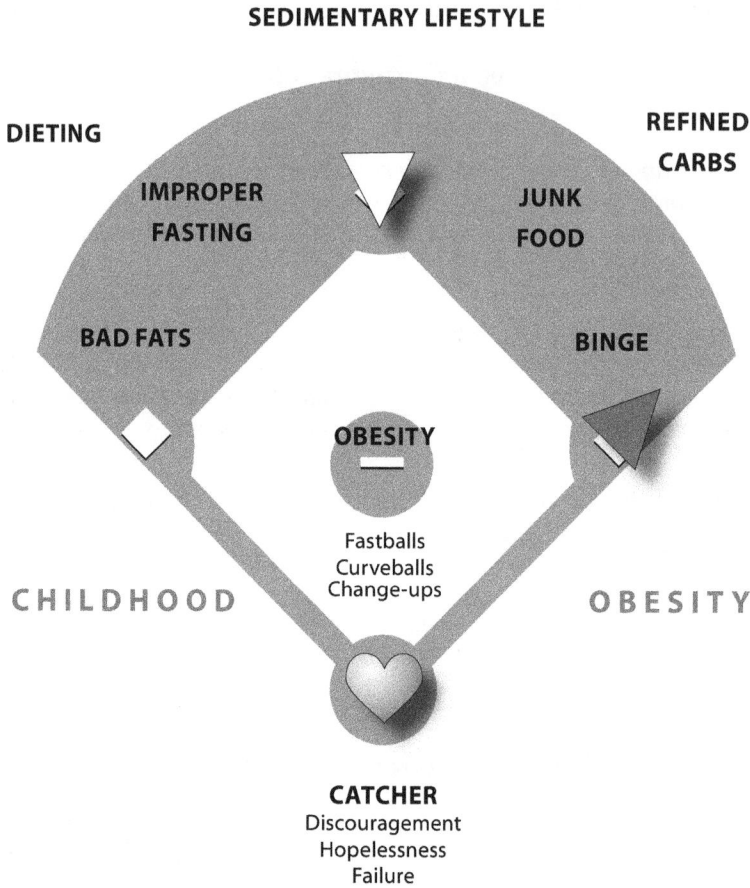

OBESITY PUZZLE

Probably the most valuable part of the Bases Loaded Program is not how it changes you or your child on the outside, but how it changes your whole family on the inside.

Conclusion

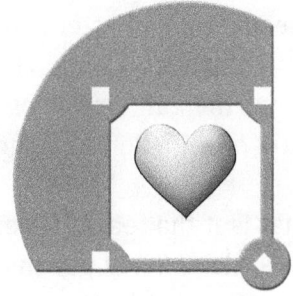

As one can see, the Obesity Puzzle is complete. We have found all the pieces and put the puzzle together. The puzzle shows a baseball field with the players of the opposing team on the field. The game is already in progress. We see Obesity with his three pitches ready and waiting. We see some of Obesity's teammates, Binge, Junk Food and Bad Fats to mention a few. We see the catcher ready to whisper words of discouragement, hopelessness and failure in the ear of the batter.

On the home side, we see that a few of the players have made hits. Nourishment Triangle is on first. Physical Activity Triangle is on second. All eyes are waiting for the next batter. Who is the next batter?

There is a strategy used in the batting order. Coaches put their good solid batters, those who consistently hit singles, up to bat in the 1,2,3 positions. We call the 4th and 5th batters power hitters because they are the ones who consistently hit doubles, triples and home runs. The strategy is to get a few players on base, then get your power hitters to get a long hit to allow teammates to score. So who are the power hitters? The power hitters are the parent and child in that order. Parent, you are up to bat.

Parent up to Bat

Baseball is a team sport. For the most part, that is true. There is a time in the game, though, when baseball becomes a truly individual test. That is when we come to bat. Baseball is the only game I know of that by design allows nine players to focus all their attention on one player of the opposing team. When a batter comes to bat it is a particularly lonely experience. The pitcher will try to manipulate the batter with skill and deception. The batter hears the voices of the other eight members of the opposing team. In particular, the catcher whispers words of discouragement and failure into the batter's ear. Does the batter feel nervous? Of course, the batter would not be normal if there was not that nervous feeling inside their stomach. Regardless of that feeling, it has to be done. Ultimately, every batter must face the test alone. Every player has to stand against the opposition alone. So it is in baseball, so it is in the battle against obesity, so it is in life.

It seems that a batter comes to home plate with nothing more than their bat and skill to prove them all wrong. They can "still" the chanting voices and get a hit if they keep their eye on the ball, and allow their body to do naturally that which has been practiced for hours on end. Perhaps, though, there is more!

What is it that each batter does before facing the opposition? They orient themselves to home plate! They get their feet right, get in position, and then tap the outside edge of home plate with their bat. Notice that, someone altered home plate into the symbol of a heart. My Aunt Dorothy used to say "There is no place like home." I agree, but how does the "heart" and the home relate in the fight against childhood obesity? To answer this question, let us go back in time to visit a home in a forgotten era.

Great Grandma Minnie

From my grandmother, I learned of my great grandmother, Minnie. She was born on the 100th year anniversary of America, July 4, 1876. Her husband was a traveling salesman, which meant that Minnie was essentially a single mom most of the time.

They lived in Dayton Ohio, not too far from the Wright Brothers' Bicycle Shop. These were the same brothers that went on to invent the first airplane. Minnie lived to be almost ninety years old. She grew up riding in a horse and buggy, and lived long enough to see men circle the planet in space capsules. Minnie witnessed all the inventions that came between these two technologies. She also witnessed lifestyle changes that occurred over the years, as America became a modern nation. My grandmother would speak wistfully of her growing up years, and the influence that her mom, Minnie, had on her life.

Those were different times. Grandma spoke of working in the garden, of nights just being with her family, reading books or listening to the radio. Family reunions, stories of cousins and aunts, all kinds of stories came from my Grandma's mouth to my ear as if these events occurred yesterday. There were stories of hardship mixed in with all these fond memories. Children and parents were close out of necessity. They had to work together to overcome the hardships. The absence of iPods, DVDs, video games, and internet, caused people back then to enrich their lives through their family. Children and parents talked about all the challenges that pertained to their lives. Along with these

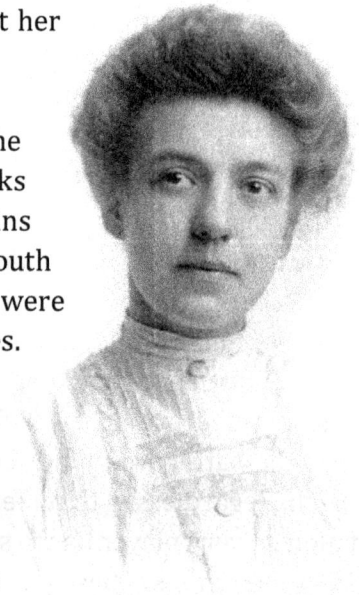

challenges, they discussed possible solutions. Children viewed their parents not only as parents, but also as older and wiser friends who passed through the same problems that they were facing. Wars, work, religion, school, sports, and the Saturday Evening Post were all topics of supplemental discussions. Meals were social events, the settings whereby these conversations happened.

Because the food was not convenient, but had to be prepared by somebody, the availability of food ended with dinner, leaving children and parents with more time together. They cleaned the dishes, continued their conversations, perhaps read together or finished any remaining chores before it was time to retire for the evening. Does all this "talk" of the past sound familiar? Unfortunately, to most of us living in the developed nations of the world, this way of life seems slightly foreign to our way of life.

The Good and Bad of Science

Science teaches; "For every action there is an opposite and equal reaction." There is much good which has come from technology and the economic prosperity associated with developed nations. Through science and technology we have conquered the elements. We can heat ourselves with natural fuel and cool ourselves with air conditioning. We have cured numerous diseases, increased life expectancy, and made life more comfortable through innovation. But what of the "opposite and equal reactions" to those advancements which we call "good?"

What are the negative consequences associated with development? Visually, if we were to represent the "loss" that occurs over time in a developed or developing nation, I believe it would look like the comparison shown in the following visual **(Figure 40)**. With development comes a demanding almost oppressive power, exerted upon the families of that nation. This power is the ability to separate and isolate. While the parts of the two families shown in this visual are the same, the hectic schedule and demands of life associated with a "developed" country have successfully destroyed the time, the overlap, and the richness of the 21st century family shown here. In this worst-case scenario, the family shares only the home they sleep in at night.

Herein we find the negative cost associated with development. The less amount of overlap that a family shares, the less strength a child has to meet the challenges the world presents. In the effort to keep up with America, many of us have tried to run faster than we have the strength to run. Running has severed us from the physical, familial, and social roots, which define us, and bind us together as human beings. It is within this context of severing and isolating that the phenomenon of childhood obesity has emerged and prospered.

Family Dynamics

19th/Early 20th Century   **Late 20th/Early 21st Century**

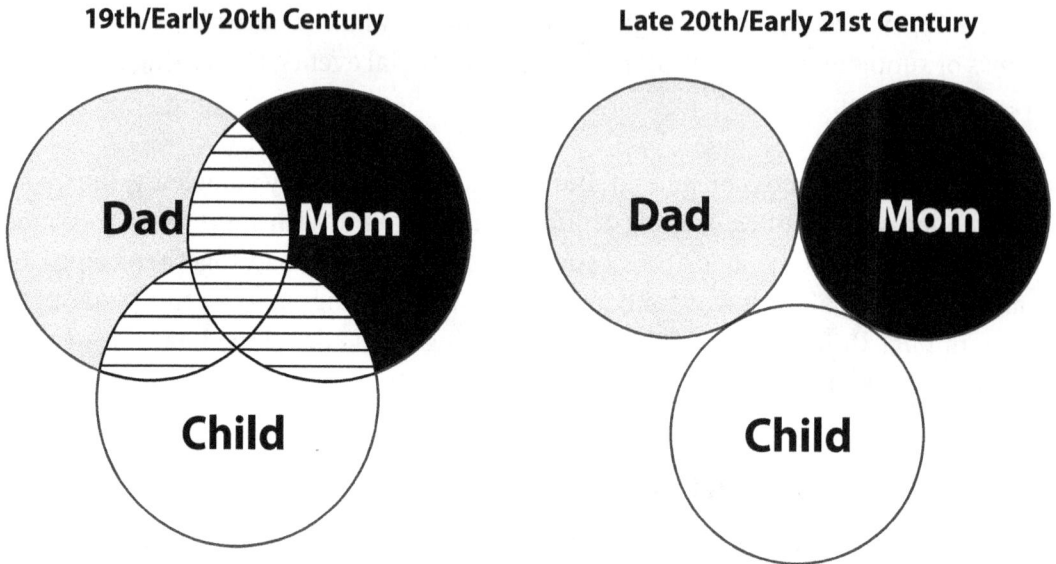

Figure 40: Family Dynamics - The hectic schedule and demands of life associated with our developed nation, have successfully destroyed the unity of the 21st century family shown here.

In the final analysis, the phenomenon of childhood obesity is only partially our fault. Parents must accept responsibility for the poor eating habits of their family. The greater part of childhood obesity, though, represents a "backlash" from development. Society and development are forces that are a mixture of both good and bad. They are forces, which, left unchecked will dominate how we manage the home. Fortunately, we as parents have the advantage. We are the home team. We have the ability to sift the good from the bad and decide "who" the boss of the home will be. Probably the most valuable part of the Bases Loaded Program is not how it changes you or your child on the outside, but how it changes your whole family on the inside. Do not be surprised if your household starts to resemble Minnie's household. There of course will be differences. Your family will continue to use the Internet and all the good things that come from science, but you will use these tools to bring your family together, and not allow these tools to isolate family members.

I must admit that my living room resembles a zoo full of strange animals and sounds when my wife and I help with the homework at night, but the family closeness and availability of parents to children is the same as Minnie's household. In both a physical and social sense, Bases Loaded is better described as a retreat to the past rather than "an advancement" of science. It is a restoration of a truly important part of human existence. It can provide healing to the heart. It can be a homecoming. Now we can answer the question posed earlier, in regards to how the "heart" and "home" relate in the fight with childhood obesity.

Playing with "Heart"

I am going to offer some advice that may seem like a contradiction. Remember how I told parents to "have fun" and "be more like a child" in an earlier chapter? Now that, you are up to bat, I am going to ask you to be an adult again. I am going to ask you to remember all those words you learned from Coach Tuff AzNails when you were involved in sports at a younger age. This game against Obesity has been a tough deadlocked battle. The difference between winning and losing in games like these is determined by something more than skill. It is determined by a matter of the heart.

Home is truly where the heart is. It is the place where we feel love. It is where children feel love. Home is where we learn love. Most parents learn that love is much more than a feeling. Love is also a conscious decision. Love involves dedication and sacrifice. It means putting others ahead of yourself and giving out more than you receive. An athlete who plays with "heart" is a player who allows the principles of selflessness to govern their actions on the playing field. They are willing to sacrifice personal recognition or glory so that their team might win.

There is something admirable in Mr. Metabolism's insistence that we human beings have not changed from being hunter/gatherers. It is an insistence that defies the bad forces of society. Development and technology have changed us on the outside, but we are no different from our ancestors. We are still the same on the inside. Human beings need one another. Children still look to parents physically, emotionally, and spiritually to meet the challenges of the world.

Children need the overlap. They need the peace within themselves so that even though they face a harsh-cruel world, they feel the answers are available and that they are not left to find the answers alone. In this respect, parents are still the hunter/gatherers for their family.

Parents are to be the source of love for their children. Children should feel loved first thing in the morning so that they do not have to go through the day in "starvation love mode." Parents must be the givers—the players who play with "heart." Each day is a new day, a new beginning, in the relationship we have with our children. We cannot expect them to survive on what we gave them, a week ago, or a month ago. We must provide that nourishment of love that brings life daily. In doing this, parents turn the grey color of a child into rainbow colors and make the journey of life into an adventure.

A wise man once taught me that children are entitled to just a few things from their parent or parents. They are entitled to food, water, clothes, and shelter from the elements. In addition, to these physical necessities, they are "entitled" to all the love that a parent can give them. Why, one might ask, is a child entitled to a parent's love? In being loved, a human being becomes capable of loving others. In receiving love, a child can grow to recognize and choose love over the counterfeits of love. In observing parents play the game of life with "heart," children also become players who play the game with "heart."

Just as, Mr. Metabolism returns a "bright burning of energy" to us when we feed him in the morning, so too, children will repay a parent's love with love in return. It will not happen in one day, but through care and nurture, the relationship will be as a small seed that grows into a beautiful plant. In addition and beyond that reciprocal love, the love can be passed down to future generations, as well. Such is the game of life! It can be a beautiful game, a game of countless "extra innings."

Who will Choose, Obesity or You?

We put the "Obesity Puzzle" together. We know the names of the opposing team's players. We understand their tactics and how they play the game. By now I think we all understand that this struggle against childhood obesity is much more than a game. It is a war! The consequences of this war are serious. Winning this war will allow children to enjoy freedom over captivity, health over sickness, and life over death. The question we as parents must face is this; "Do we want to continue fighting this war according to Obesity's rules, or do we want to be in command of the situation?" There is no middle ground here. If we shrug shoulders and do not make a decision, then we automatically give back to Obesity the power to choose. What will Obesity choose? Obesity will make sure children spend their time in front of the TV. Obesity will feed them food that is fast and convenient for us, but unhealthy. Instead of finding comfort from concerned parents, Obesity will compel children to search for comfort in junk food or find diversion in a virtual world. We as parents have the ability to change things within the family. That is the starting place for society. It is in the hearts of parents. It is our hope that Bases Loaded will help families on that path that leads to health, fun, love, and happiness, to allow them to "run and not be weary, to walk and not faint."

A New Beginning

Discouragement is one of Obesity's greatest tools. In the battle against Obesity, let us remember Mr. Metabolism's philosophy. Each day is a new beginning, a new day, a new time up to bat. Do not be frustrated, if your child occasionally has a day where they make a strike instead of a hit. Joe had such days. Look at Joe's weight chart to see a good example. Notice how much weight Joe gained after Halloween 2005. Guess what happened? Joe went out for Halloween, ate a bunch of candy at the end of the night, then he went to sleep.

The important thing about this example is that Joe learned from the experience. He came back up to bat. Strikes are never a bad thing if one keeps their mind and heart on the big picture. In regards to childhood obesity, the big picture is this; "We now have the principles that empower us, to transform the lives of our children for good!"

Your Child is Up to Bat

Your child approaches the plate. Here is the great part; In the Bases Loaded Plan, there is no such thing as the rule, "Three strikes and you are out." Through patience, diligence, and even strikes, your child will succeed. As surely as the sun rises in the morning, so too, your son or daughter will awake to a new life!

Parent, your time at bat has provided the critical hit needed to load the bases. Your child is now at bat and waits for the pitch. It is right where they like it, "down the middle."

Your child connects with the ball, and sees a glimpse of it and starts running to first base. The ball is way above the right fielder. The center fielder runs over to help chase it down as it lands at the edge of the field and rolls towards the parking lot.

Your child approaches second base and looks to see the outfielders still chasing the ball. The third base coach waves his arms and motions your child towards home.

Your child rounds third, and sees teammates waiting at home plate. Family members on the home team side, clap and cheer. Everyone on the team surrounds your child when home plate is finally tagged. The journey around the bases has brought your child back to where they were before, but somehow they

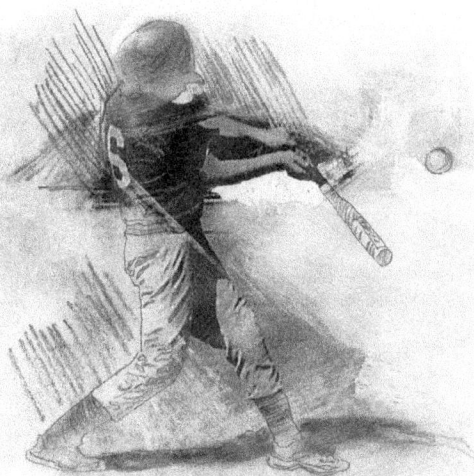

are not the same as before. Your mighty batter has hit a grand slam and won a deadlocked game. Teammates hoist their hero on their shoulders and make their way to the family. All of you clap and cheer and hug each other with joy!

At the end of the night when all is said and done, sleep yields one more time to the excitement of the day as you say goodnight. Eventually, the family hero starts to fade. Somewhere between this world and the unconscious, a rhyme floats into their mind. At first the words seem foreign, but soon familiar as if coming from deep within the soul. The words come with joy, and like a lullaby, the words carry our hero to the world of happy dreams, to relive the moments of the day, once again.

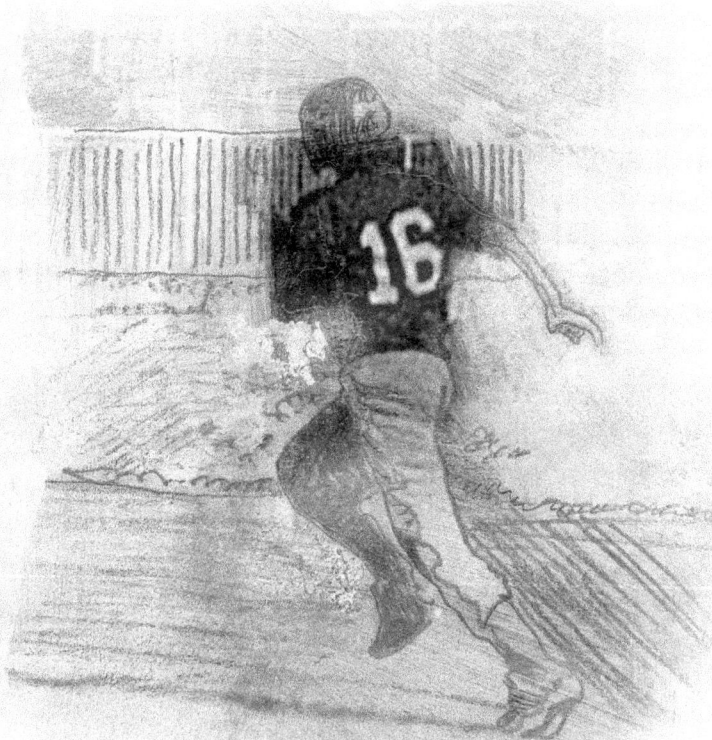

Life is good

Life is worth the living

Today is good

Tomorrow is a new day

Life is worth the giving

Endnotes

[1] Neergaard, Lauran, *Obesity Leads to Rocketing Health Spending,* (Salt Lake City: Deseret News, Sec. A, July 28, 2009): 3.

[2] Ibid., 3.

[3] Simopoulos, Artemis P., and Robinson, J., *The Omega Diet,* (New York: Harper Collins Publishers, 1999): 24.

[4] Neergaard, Lauran, *Obesity Leads to Rocketing Health Spending,* (Salt Lake City: Deseret News, Sec. A, July 28, 2009): 3.

[5] Cooper, Robert K., and Cooper, L., L., *Flip the Switch,* (New York: Rodale, 2005): 142.

[6] Ibid., 202.

[7] Ibid., 143.

[8] Simopoulos, Artemis P., and Robinson, J., *The Omega Diet,* (New York: Harper Collins Publishers, 1999): 24.

[9] Cooper, Robert K., and Cooper, L., L., *Flip the Switch,* (New York: Rodale, 2005): 58.

[10] Ibid., 57.

[11] Phillips, Bill, *Body for Life,* (New York: Harper Collins Publishers, 1999): 43.

[12] Simopoulos, Artemis P., and Robinson, J., *The Omega Diet,* (New York: Harper Collins Publishers, 1999): 24.

[13] Phillips, Bill, *Body for Life,* (New York: Harper Collins Publishers, 1999): 47.

[14] Ibid., 48.

[15] Groves, Lana, *Weighing in on Fad Diets,* (Salt Lake City: Deseret News, Sec. B, May 25, 2009): 3.

[16] Phillips, Bill, *Body for Life,* (New York: Harper Collins Publishers, 1999): 46.

[17] Balch, James F., and Balch, Phyllis A., *Prescription for Nutritional Healing,* Second Ed., (New York: Avery Publishing Group, 1997): 228

[18] Ibid., 3.

[19] Simopoulos, Artemis P., and Robinson, J., *The Omega Diet,* (New York: Harper Collins Publishers, 1999): 26.

[20] Ibid., 26.

[21] Ibid., 5.

[22] Ibid., 25.

[23] Cooper, Robert K., and Cooper, L., L., *Flip the Switch*, (New York: Rodale, 2005): 235.

[24] Simopoulos, Artemis P., and Robinson, J., *The Omega Diet,* (New York: Harper Collins Publishers, 1999): 5.

[25] Phillips, Bill, *Body for Life*, (New York: Harper Collins Publishers, 1999): 47.

[26] Brand-Miller, J., Wolever, T., M., S., Colagiuri, S., Foster-Powell, K., *The Glucose Revolution,* (New York: Marlowe & Company, 1996, 1998, 1999): 5.

[27] Ibid., 7.

[28] Cooper, Robert K., and Cooper, L., L., *Flip the Switch,* (New York: Rodale, 2005): 231.

[29] Brand-Miller, J., Wolever, T., M., S., Colagiuri, S., Foster-Powell, K., *The Glucose Revolution,* (New York: Marlowe & Company, 1996, 1998, 1999): 43.

[30] Balch, James F., and Balch, Phyllis A., *Prescription for Nutritional Healing,* Second Ed., (New York: Avery Publishing Group, 1997): 87.

[31] Ibid., 87.

[32] Ibid., 87.

[33] Brand-Miller, J., Wolever, T., M., S., Colagiuri, S., Foster-Powell, K., *The Glucose Revolution*, (New York: Marlowe & Company, 1996, 1998, 1999): 158.

[34] Ibid., 159.

[35] Balch, James F. , and Balch, Phyllis A. , *Prescription for Nutritional Healing, Second Ed. ,* (New York: Avery Publishing Group, 1997): 231.

[36] Ibid. , 231.

[37] Ibid. , 44.

[38] Hudson, Valerie, *Rethinking Cystic Fibrosis Pathology: the Critical Role of Abnormal Reduced Glutathione (GSH) Transport caused by CFTR Mutation,* (Free Radical Biology & Medicine, Vol. 30, No. 12, 200 : 1451.

[39] Balch, James F. , and Balch, Phyllis A. , *Prescription for Nutritional Healing, Second Ed. ,* (New York: Avery Publishing Group, 1997): 39.

[40] Ibid. , 44.

[41] Ibid. , 44.

[42] Ibid. , 44.

[43] Hudson, Valerie, *Rethinking Cystic Fibrosis Pathology: the Critical Role of Abnormal Reduced Glutathione (GSH) Transport caused by CFTR Mutation,* (Free Radical Biology & Medicine, Vol. 30, No. 12, 200 : 1441.

[44] Balch, James F. , and Balch, Phyllis A. , *Prescription for Nutritional Healing, Second Ed. ,* (New York: Avery Publishing Group, 1997): 44.

[45] Ibid. , 44.

[46] Ibid. , 39.

[47] Hudson, Valerie, *Rethinking Cystic Fibrosis Pathology: the Critical Role of Abnormal Reduced Glutathione (GSH) Transport caused by CFTR Mutation,* (Free Radical Biology & Medicine,

Vol. 30, No. 12, 200 : 1442.

[48] Ibid. , 1442.

[49] Ibid. , 1451.

[50] Balch, James F. , and Balch, Phyllis A. , *Prescription for Nutritional Healing, Second Ed. *, (New York: Avery Publishing Group, 1997): 37. [35] Balch, James F. , and Balch, Phyllis A. , *Prescription for Nutritional Healing, Second Ed. *, (New York: Avery Publishing Group, 1997): 231.

[36] Ibid. , 231.

[37] Ibid. , 44.

[38] Hudson, Valerie, *Rethinking Cystic Fibrosis Pathology: the Critical Role of Abnormal Reduced Glutathione (GSH) Transport caused by CFTR Mutation*, (Free Radical Biology & Medicine, Vol. 30, No. 12, 200 : 1451.

[39] Balch, James F. , and Balch, Phyllis A. , *Prescription for Nutritional Healing, Second Ed. *, (New York: Avery Publishing Group, 1997): 39.

[40] Ibid. , 44.

[41] Ibid. , 44.

[42] Ibid. , 44.

[43] Hudson, Valerie, *Rethinking Cystic Fibrosis Pathology: the Critical Role of Abnormal Reduced Glutathione (GSH) Transport caused by CFTR Mutation*, (Free Radical Biology & Medicine, Vol. 30, No. 12, 200 : 1441.

[44] Balch, James F. , and Balch, Phyllis A. , *Prescription for Nutritional Healing, Second Ed. *, (New York: Avery Publishing Group, 1997): 44.

[45] Ibid. , 44.

[46] Ibid. , 39.

[47] Hudson, Valerie, *Rethinking Cystic Fibrosis Pathology: the Critical Role of Abnormal Reduced Glutathione (GSH) Transport caused by CFTR Mutation*, (Free Radical Biology & Medicine, Vol. 30, No. 12, 200 : 1442.

[48] Ibid. , 1442.

[49] Ibid. , 1451.

[50] Balch, James F. , and Balch, Phyllis A. , *Prescription for Nutritional Healing, Second Ed. ,* (New York: Avery Publishing Group, 1997): 37. [51] Cooper, Robert K., and Cooper, L., L., *Flip the Switch,* (New York: Rodale, 2005): 143.

[52] Balch, James F., and Balch, Phyllis A., *Prescription for Nutritional Healing, Second Ed.,* (New York: Avery Publishing Group, 1997): 548.

[53] Cooper, Robert K., and Cooper, L., L., *Flip the Switch,* (New York: Rodale, 2005): 48.

[54] Groves, Lana, *Weighing in on Fad Diets,* (Salt Lake City: Deseret News, Sec. B, May 25, 2009): 3.

[55] Phillips, Bill, *Body for Life,* (New York: Harper Collins Publishers, 1999): 43.

[56] Ibid., 43-44.

[57] Cooper, Robert K., and Cooper, L., L., *Flip the Switch,* (New York: Rodale, 2005): 148.

[58] Ibid., 143.

[59] Cloud, John, *Why Exercise Won't Make You Thin,* (Time Magazine, http://www.com/time/health/article/0,8599,1914857,00, Sec. 4, Aug. 9, 2009): 1

[60] Ibid., Sec. 3, pp. 2.

[61] Ibid., Sec. 1, pp. 1.

[62] Cooper, Robert K., and Cooper, L., L., *Flip the Switch,* (New York: Rodale, 2005): 166.

[63] Cloud, John, *Why Exercise Won't Make You Thin,* (Time Magazine, http://www.com/time/health/article/0,8599,1914857,00, Sec.1, Aug. 9, 2009): 2.

[64]Peck, Scott, *The Road Less Traveled,* (New York: Simon & Schuster, 1978): 243.

[65] Ibid., 280-281.

[66] Ibid., 283.

[67] Ibid., 283.

[68] Cooper, Robert K., and Cooper, L., L., *Flip the Switch,* (New York: Rodale, 2005): 68.

[69] Cloud, John, *Why Exercise Won't Make You Thin,* (Time Magazine, http://www.com/time/health/article/0,8599,1914857,00, Sec.3, Aug. 9, 2009): 3.

[70] Ibid., 3.

www.ingramcontent.com/pod-product-compliance
Lightning Source LLC
Chambersburg PA
CBHW080330270326
41927CB00014B/3155